MEET
YOUR
BACTERIA

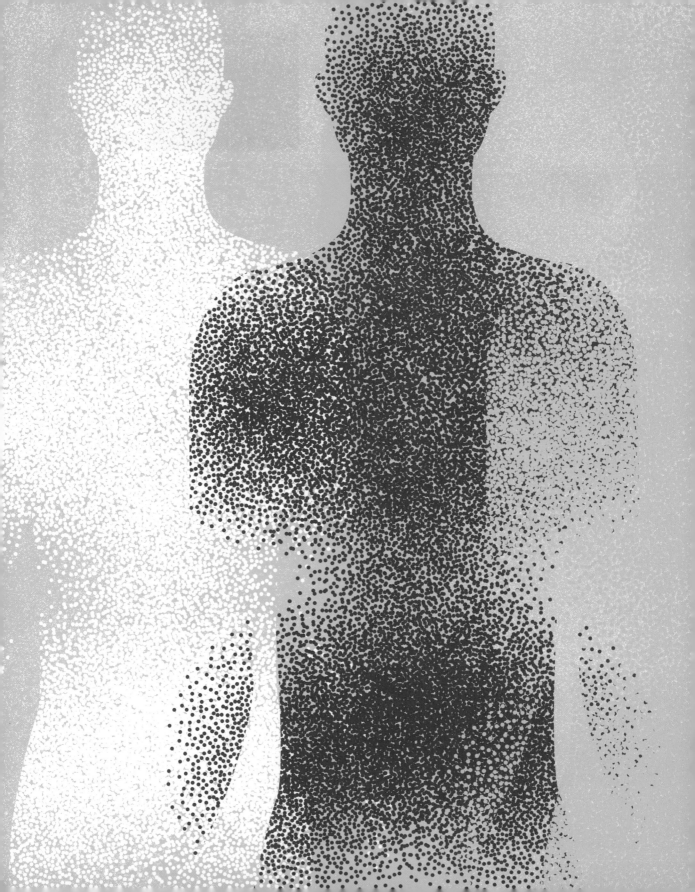

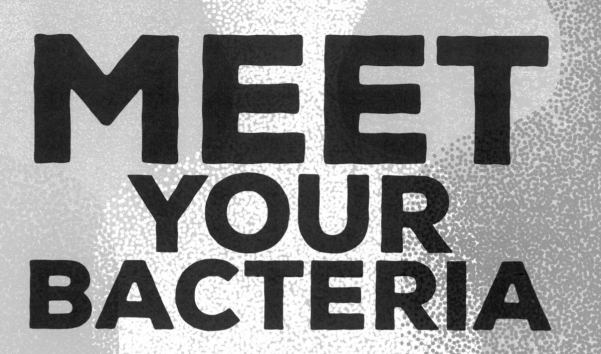

MEET YOUR BACTERIA

FOREWORD BY
Professor Glenn Gibson

**NICOLA TEMPLE &
CATHERINE WHITLOCK**

FIREFLY BOOKS

A FIREFLY BOOK

Published by Firefly Books Ltd. 2018

First printing

Publisher Cataloging-in-Publication Data (U.S.)

Library of Congress Control Number: 2018934532

Library and Archives Canada Cataloguing in Publication

Temple, Nicola, author
    Meet your bacteria : the hidden communities that live in
your gut & other organs / Nicola Temple & Catherine Whitlock ;
foreword by Professor Glenn Gibson.
Includes bibliographical references and index.
ISBN 978-0-228-10126-0 (softcover)

    1. Bacteria--Popular works. 2. Human body--Microbiology--
Popular works. I. Whitlock, Catherine, author II. Gibson, Glenn
R., writer of foreword III. Title.
QR74.8.T44 2018   579.3   C2018-901142-4

Published in the United States by   Published in Canada by
Firefly Books (U.S.) Inc.   Firefly Books Ltd.
P.O. Box 1338, Ellicott Station   50 Staples Avenue, Unit 1
Buffalo, New York 14205   Richmond Hill, Ontario L4B 0A7

Printed and bound in China

First published by Cassell, a division of   Edited and designed by JMS Books LLP
Octopus Publishing Group Ltd, Carmelite House   & Wayne Blades
50 Victoria Embankment   Illustrations by Tonwen Jones
London EC4Y 0DZ

PUBLISHING DIRECTOR Trevor Davies
ASSISTANT EDITOR Ellie Corbett
SENIOR DESIGNER Jaz Bahra
SENIOR PRODUCTION MANAGER Peter Hunt

For our respective families:
Shelby and Morgan
Paul, James, Mary and Thomas

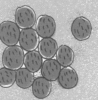

Disclaimer/Publisher's note
All reasonable care has been taken in the preparation of this book but the information it contains is not intended as a substitute for expert medical
advice and you must seek professional advice if you are in any doubt about any medical condition. Any application of the ideas and information
contained in this book is at the reader's sole discretion and risk. Before making any changes in your health regime, always consult a doctor.

Photos of bacteria
Some of the greatly magnified images of bacteria in the book are electron micrographs: a photograph or computer-enhanced image of a specimen
taken using an electron microscope. These immensely powerful microscopes magnify bacteria 100–250 thousand times, compared with the maximum
magnification of a standard light microscope of one thousand.

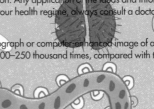

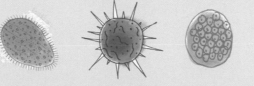

CONTENTS

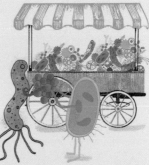

FOREWORD

Whether we like it not, we all have trillions and trillions of bacteria living in or on our bodies. Actually, we should like it: these inhabitants do us a lot of good, with our lives being impossible without them. So, while humans may be the ultimate "hotel," our guests make a really positive contribution to well-being. I have been researching human gut bacteria for 30 years now, never dreaming that this topic would become as popular and widely studied as it is today. Indeed, the general recognition that not all bacteria are bad is in itself a major achievement.

Many articles claim that the human microbiome is a new and emerging research area. For obvious reasons, I cannot agree with this; however, the field has never been so important or better understood, nor has it ever offered such potential for future scientific progress. Several microbiomes are associated with our bodies, and their contribution to health and disease is undoubted. The really good news is that each of these ecosystems is amenable to change that can help improve interactions with the host (that's you). This is a crucial way to improve our health. The number of issues that can be tackled is truly startling.

Gastroenteritis, ulcerative colitis, Crohn's disease, obesity, autism, certain cancers, anxiety, depression, metabolic syndrome, diabetes, coronary heart disease, tooth decay, acne, eczema, asthma, recurrent thrush, urogenital infections, irritable bowel syndrome and antibiotic-associated diarrhea are all on the research agenda — and even that is not an exhaustive list.

Interventions are constantly being researched, tested and produced to improve the human microbiota composition, and thereby health status. In many cases this involves "germ warfare" in its simplest sense: pathogenic microbes involved in the onset and/or maintenance of a disorder being subverted or inhibited by fortifying a more beneficial community. Fortunately, our microbiome (unlike our genetics) is flexible and can be changed. To this end, probiotics, prebiotics and synbiotics are all popular. Robust and confirmed products offer zero to negligible risk — an almost unique selling point in terms of therapeutic intervention. The efficacy and application of these products has been propelled by a much-improved understanding of the microbiome community. This was a direct result of the "molecular revolution" in the late 1990s, which provided reliable and efficient tools for monitoring human microbiota.

Nearly two decades later, we are in a similar phase with the "metabolic revolution." Today, our far greater understanding of microbiome functionality is being coupled with trials that assess not only microbial composition but also health biomarkers, patients' symptoms and reduced disease risk. Many 21st-century ailments will undergo far better management than has hitherto been the case. This may be achieved through interventions that are safe, user-friendly and reliable. These are extremely exciting times.

This brings me to *Meet Your Bacteria*. It is now imperative that consumers, healthcare workers, product manufacturers and other interested communities are given an understandable yet scientifically accurate assessment of the current state of the art, or indeed of the science, its current research and findings. This excellent book for the general reader should help to stimulate interest and propel their use and application. Now is the time to push forward with

Bacteria in the spotlight

approaches that will help many people, and have an impact on us all. *Meet Your Bacteria* makes a significant contribution toward pulling the relevant disciplines together, necessary to appreciate the full potential of these microbial inhabitants. I hope you enjoy reading this terrific study of what is arguably the most important health and medical challenge of modern times.

PROFESSOR GLENN GIBSON

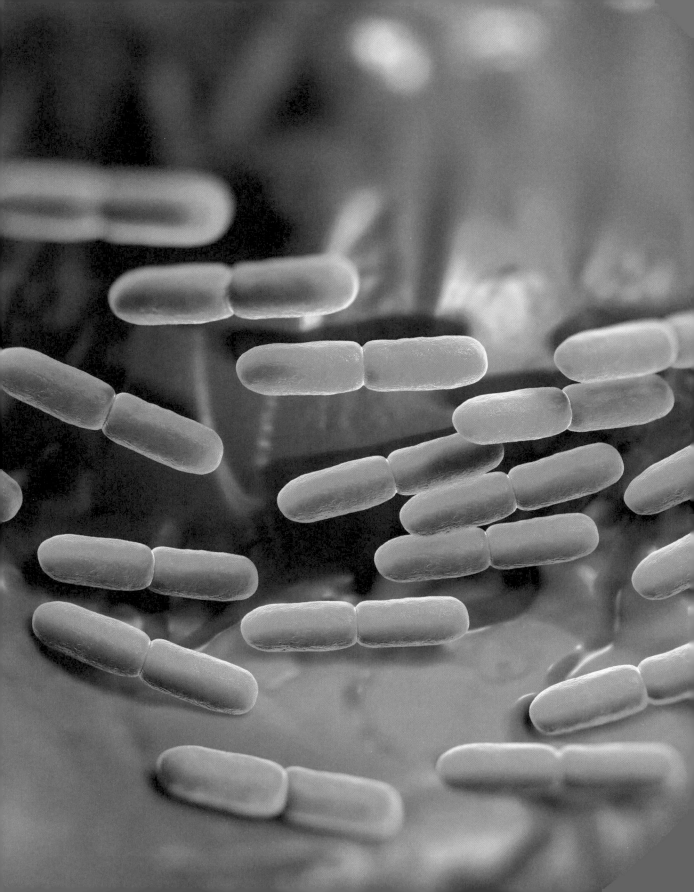

CHAPTER ONE

WHAT HAVE BACTERIA EVER DONE FOR US?

Bacteria affect every aspect of our lives on a daily basis. The bacteria that live in and on your body help you to digest food, protect you from harmful microbes and even contribute to your mental well-being. However, less friendly bacteria can also cause a variety of illnesses from sore throats to serious, even life-threatening diseases. It is bacteria that help to ripen flavorful cheeses, ferment cocoa and convert sugars into alcohol — but they can also cause foods to decay and give us food poisoning.

On a much broader scale, bacteria help to decompose organic matter, working like an efficient recycling center to break down material and return nutrients back into the earth. They also turn carbon and nitrogen in the atmosphere into forms that plants and animals can use. Quite simply, we wouldn't be here if it weren't for bacteria. This chapter explores these amazing organisms, from what they are and what they look like to how they interact with us as their hosts.

Lactobacillus **bacteria.**

INTRODUCING YOUR GUESTS

Your body is home to trillions of microorganisms, or microbes: living organisms too small for us to see without a microscope. Most of them are bacteria and each one is a single cell, the smallest unit of life.

There are enough bacteria living on the average person to fill a can of soup. The number of bacterial cells on our bodies may outnumber our human cells by 3:1 (estimates actually range from 10:1 to 1:1). But bacteria are not the only microorganisms to call your body home. Other microbes — such as archaea, protozoa, viruses and fungi — live there too. This community of microbes is called your "microbiome," and it is unique to every individual.

HOW MANY?

Your body is made of about 30 trillion human cells, but the cells of all the organisms that make up your microbiome are far more numerous. Your mouth is home to around 500 different species of bacteria alone, while an estimated 100 trillion bacteria live in your gut.

WHAT DO MICROBES DO?

Microbes infamously cause diseases — and we refer to these less pleasant microbes as germs. Viruses, the smallest and simplest of the microorganisms, cause illnesses such as the common cold and flu. Bacteria cause infections, for example strep throat and tuberculosis. Athlete's foot and candidiasis (thrush) are among the common fungal infections, while protozoan infections include malaria and giardiasis. To avoid these germs, many people try to keep themselves and their environments as clean and germ-free as possible. However, only a tiny fraction of the microorganisms that live on and inside you are actually harmful. Most members of your microbial community are either completely benign or actively beneficial.

For example, some bacteria help to train and maintain your immune system; others manufacture vitamins or supply other vital nutrients; while yet others proliferate harmlessly, preventing more harmful species from becoming established simply by crowding them out physically. So it is essential to maintain a healthy, balanced microbiome. The over-prescription of antibiotics, the use of hand sanitizers and the decrease in time spent outside in "dirty" environments are all aspects of our modern world that have contributed to dramatic changes in the microbes that colonize human beings. These changes have been implicated in the global rise of autoimmune disorders, such as eczema and Crohn's disease, as well as obesity, cancer and depression. The message is, we mess with our microbiome at our peril.

GET TO KNOW YOUR GROUPINGS

The following terms are frequently used to refer to different groups of the microorganisms living in and on your body:

BACTERIUM:
the singular form of bacteria, referring to a single cell (see pages 14–15)

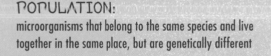

POPULATION:
microorganisms that belong to the same species and live together in the same place, but are genetically different

COLONY:
a group of genetically identical bacteria, known as clones

COMMUNITY:
microorganisms that belong to different species but live together in the same place

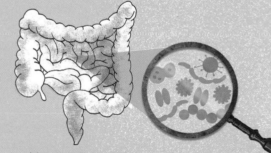

MICROBIOME:
all the microorganisms, with their combined genome, that exist in a particular environment

MICROBES ON THE EVOLUTIONARY TREE

Your microbiome consists of microorganisms from many different branches of the evolutionary tree that scientists use to understand relationships between all living organisms. Despite coming from diverse and distantly related groups, these microbes have all found ways to survive and thrive in the different habitats your body provides.

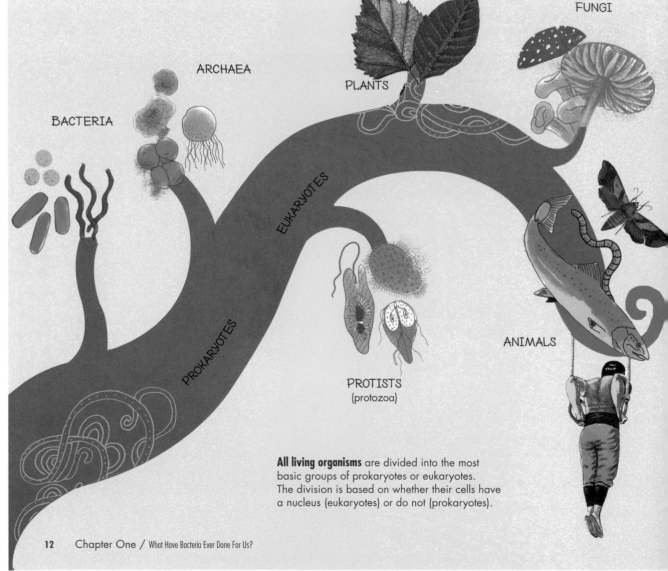

FUNGI

ARCHAEA

PLANTS

BACTERIA

EUKARYOTES

PROKARYOTES

PROTISTS
(protozoa)

ANIMALS

All living organisms are divided into the most basic groups of prokaryotes or eukaryotes. The division is based on whether their cells have a nucleus (eukaryotes) or do not (prokaryotes).

The first organisms on Earth were prokaryotes. They appeared roughly 4 billion years ago and are the ancestors of all living things. Their cell structure is very simple, with no nucleus nor any membrane-bound compartments. In other cells these compartments, known as organelles, keep all the enzymes, proteins and other compounds needed to carry out specific functions in the cell in one place. A bacterium, which has no organelles, keeps everything it needs distributed throughout the cell — about as efficient as keeping spices all over the house rather than together in a spice rack. However, this lack of efficiency has not prevented prokaryotes from thriving in every habitat on Earth including the human body.

ARCHAEA, NOT BACTERIA

Scientists originally thought that all prokaryotes were bacteria, noting that some seemed to have an affinity for extreme habitats, such as hot springs and salt lakes. Closer investigation revealed that some of these extreme "bacteria" had features that were quite distinct; they were, in fact, more similar to eukaryotes. So in 1977 these organisms were moved into their own group of single-celled prokaryotes, known as archaea. Not all archaea live in extreme habitats: they are found in the ocean and soil, for example, as well as in the human body. There are as yet no known disease-causing archaea, but scientists have only recently started to study these members of the human microbiome.

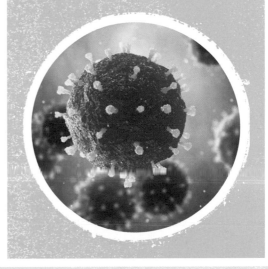

WHERE ARE VIRUSES?

Viruses do not fit very neatly under the existing classification system: whether they are living organisms or not is still under debate. Scientists have placed them in their own classification system while investigations continue.

Viruses contain genetic material and evolve, but they don't have a cellular structure and need a host to reproduce.

PROTOZOA AND FUNGI

These organisms are both found in the human microbiome and are eukaryotes, containing a nucleus and other organelles. Protozoa are single-celled organisms and many of them are parasitic, making their role in a healthy human microbiome still unclear. The microscopic fungi that we host are usually multi-cellular; nobody is fungus-free, but fungi are found in far fewer numbers than bacteria. For this reason we will now concentrate on the most abundant and diverse of your guests ... bacteria.

IDENTIFYING YOUR GUESTS

Although bacteria are relatively simple organisms, usually no more than a few micrometers (a few millionths of a meter or inch) in length, they come in a variety of shapes and sizes, and group together in several different ways. Scientists use these obvious physical features to identify and classify bacteria.

STANDARD FEATURES

DNA: A singular circular chromosome, tangled within the cell, which contains all the genes this cell needs to live.

CELL MEMBRANE: A semi-permeable membrane that separates the interior of the cell from the exterior.

CELL WALL: The rigid outer layer of the cell. It not only provides physical support, but also protects the cell from damage

CYTOPLASM: The interior environment of the cell.

RIBOSOME: The site where proteins are assembled from the genetic code.

OPTIONAL FEATURES

PLASMIDS: Small circular molecules of DNA that bacteria pick up from the environment, viruses or other bacteria. These small packets of extra DNA can really improve the cell's performance, particularly when they contain genes for antibiotic resistance or rapid growth.

FLAGELLA: Whip-like tails made of protein, used by some species for enhanced mobility.

CAPSULE: Sometimes a cell wall simply does not offer enough protection in harsh conditions. A layer made of sugar-like molecules (polysaccharides) provides extra protection.

FIMBRIAE: Hair-like structures that really help the cell stick to surfaces, for example to human cells.

THE THREE MAIN MODELS

Bacteria are grouped into one of three shapes: rods, spirals or spheres. A bacterium's shape is usually indicated in the species name. For example, the bacteria responsible for throat and ear infection is coccus-shaped, or spherical, and therefore has the name *Streptococcus* (giving us the term "strep throat" for the common infection).

The shape of a bacterium is adapted to where it lives and what it does. Due to their shape, small spherical bacteria can pack together tightly and divide more rapidly. A rod shape is better suited for bacteria that need to move, and a spiral shape is perfect for moving through thick, viscous liquids. *Campylobacter jejuni*, for example, causes food poisoning by corkscrewing through the mucus layer that lines your gut to reach the cells beneath. Bacteria can respond to changes in their environment by changing shape. They grow larger to avoid being eaten by predatory protozoa, for example, or become smaller if nutrients are limited.

RODS
(bacillus)

SPIRALS
(including vibrios, spirilla
and spirochaetes)

SPHERES
(coccus)

BACTERIAL CELL

The basic components of a bacterium and other features that it may possess.

1. CELL WALL	6. CAPSULE
2. CELL MEMBRANE	7. PLASMID
3. DNA	8. FIMBRIA
4. CYTOPLASM	9. FLAGELLUM
5. RIBOSOME	

EVERY BACTERIUM COMES EQUIPPED WITH STOCK FEATURES ESSENTIAL TO KEEP THE CELL RUNNING. HOWEVER, CERTAIN SPECIES ALSO HAVE OPTIONAL FEATURES THAT CAN REALLY IMPROVE THEIR PERFORMANCE

SHAPE SHIFTERS

The bacteria responsible for urinary tract infections (*Escherichia coli*) changes shape at different stages of an infection. These changes in shape make it easier for the bacteria to multiply and spread within the urinary tract. In this police-style "line-up" (1) is a single, non-motile (not capable of movement), rod-shaped *E. coli* 2 hours after infection; (2) is a non-motile, coccus-shaped *E. coli,* found in a large group about 7 hours after infection; (3) is a motile, rod-shaped *E. coli* that broke away from the group around 12 or more hours after infection.

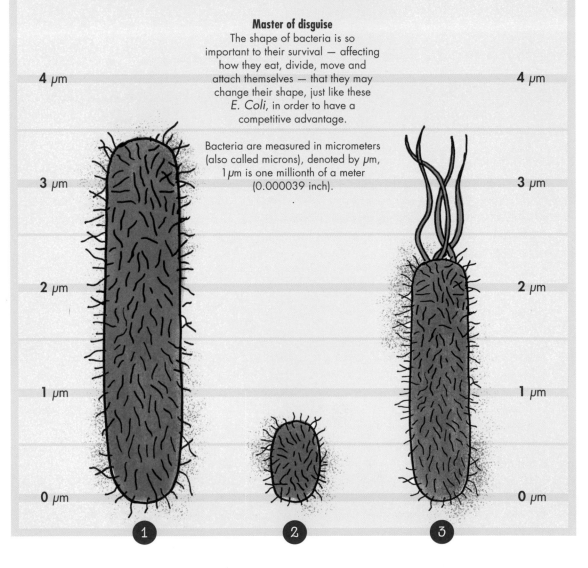

Master of disguise
The shape of bacteria is so important to their survival — affecting how they eat, divide, move and attach themselves — that they may change their shape, just like these *E. Coli,* in order to have a competitive advantage.

Bacteria are measured in micrometers (also called microns), denoted by *μm*, 1 *μm* is one millionth of a meter (0.000039 inch).

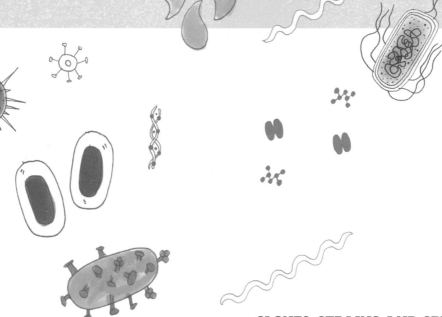

ON THE MOVE

Many, but not all, species of bacteria are able to move actively in their environment. Some species have a single flagellum or a cluster of flagella, used like a propeller to push or pull the bacterium along. Spiral bacteria simply rotate to drive themselves through their environment. Some species glide across surfaces over a thick layer of slime, while others use hook-like appendages to pull themselves along.

GETTING TOGETHER

Some types of bacteria tend to gather together in pairs, groups or long chains. Even species that do not typically hang out together in groups may do so to avoid predators or harmful chemicals. Under certain circumstances, bacteria can form a complex matrix known as a biofilm. Using different types of proteins, individual cells first glue themselves firmly to a surface and then cement themselves to other bacteria cells nearby. The whole colony then encases itself in a protein shell, making it thousands of times more resistant to antibiotics than the individual cells.

CLONES, STRAINS AND SPECIES

The three terms explained below are often used to define bacteria.

CLONES: The daughter cells that come from a single bacterium through fission (see pages 28–29). They are genetically identical to the original cell. A group of clones is known as a colony.

A STRAIN OF BACTERIA: A subtype where a genetic variation has made the bacterium a little different from the rest of its species — for instance, more virulent. All the bacterium's descendants will have that variation in common, which means that they all belong to the same strain.

A SPECIES OF BACTERIA: A collection of strains with a common origin — more similar to one another than to other strains. Bacteria are rather more complicated when it comes to species. They evolve at such a tremendous rate that something which is now a new strain might, in only a few decades, have become different enough to be considered a new species. The study of bacteria just requires a more fluid concept of species than we are accustomed to.

THE GOOD, THE BAD AND THE OPPORTUNISTIC

Your microbiome is just like any other diverse community — it has its upstanding citizens and its troublemakers. While the vast majority of your bacteria are good, certain others will cause trouble, given the chance.

The "good" bacteria that make up the majority of your microbial community, such as *Lactobacillus acidophillus*, are called non-pathogens because they are not known to cause human disease. "Bad" bacteria such as *Mycobacterium tuberculosis*, the species responsible for tuberculosis, are called pathogens because they are known agents of disease — they are not members of your microbiome, but they are able to infect you. However, there are also a number of species, known as opportunistic pathogens, that can change from being peaceful members of your microbial community into downright hooligans if the opportunity arises.

WHAT OPPORTUNITY?

A number of things can happen to create the right environment for an opportunistic pathogen to thrive. A cut to the skin, for example, creates an entry point for bacteria to access tissues they

A bacterium that is beneficial in one area of the body can become troublesome if it migrates and takes hold in another area. Staphylococcus aureus is beneficial in the blue areas (right), yet harmful in those colored red.

cannot normally reach. A more serious wound, particularly one that breaches the wall of the gut, could allow bacteria to pass into the bloodstream, from where they can move to infect other areas of the body.

Opportunistic pathogens also take advantage when the immune system is compromised. This may be as a result of antibiotics, pregnancy, immune disease, malnutrition, medical procedures such as chemotherapy or even something as simple as fatigue. In these circumstances, the bad bacteria have less chance of being caught and then destroyed.

STRONG COMMUNITY
While the immune system plays an important role in policing bad bacteria, it has become increasingly clear that a strong, healthy community of microbes is equally important in inhibiting infection. Just as thriving communities of people do not tolerate bad behavior in their neighborhood, a

healthy microbiome can help to prevent infection. The microbial community uses a host of different strategies to deter troublemakers. They occupy all the space and use all the nutrients, making it physically difficult for bad bacteria to find a place to squat and find something to eat, so they simply move on. Good bacteria can change their environment to make it better suited to their needs and less suited to the needs of bad bacteria (see page 25). Good bacteria even produce toxins that inhibit the growth of bad bacteria. If none of these other strategies work, the good bacteria can also call upon the body's immune cells to help get rid of the bad guys (see page 34).

THE OPPORTUNIST:
STAPHYLOCOCCUS AUREUS
Description:
- **Coccus-shaped**
- **Found in groups**
- **Less than 1 micron in diameter**

Note: People who have Staphylococcus aureus as part of their normal microbiome (known as carriers) are more prone to infections by this bacterium. However, such infections tend to be less severe than those of non-carriers who become infected by it.

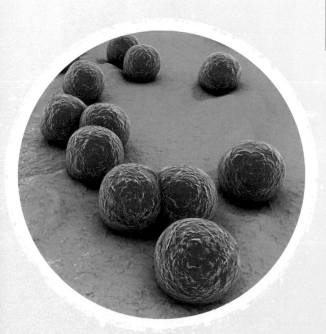

Staphylococcus aureus is usually a mild-mannered member of the human microbiome, found on the skin, in the gut and in the upper respiratory tract of about 30 percent of people. However, if there is a wound in the skin, it seizes the opportunity to prosper. Special features of its cell wall help this bacterium to attach to the proteins that form during the blood clotting process. There it can start to reproduce rapidly and wreak havoc with the immune system that is trying to repair the damaged tissue.

IN A RELATIONSHIP

The long-term relationship you have with the microorganisms in your microbiome is known as symbiosis (from sym–, meaning "together," and –biosis, meaning "living"). Many different kinds of symbiotic relationships exist in nature, from the beneficial to the harmful. Some occur between organisms of the same species, while others are between very different species, as is the case with you and your microbiome.

Symbiosis can be classified into three broad categories: mutualism, parasitism and commensalism. These terms are used throughout this book as we explore some of the key players in the human microbiome.

Humans and dogs are two different species that enjoy a mutually beneficial relationship.

MUTUALISM

A symbiotic relationship that is beneficial to both species. For example, the first species may provide a safe place for the second to thrive, while the second may provide vital nutrients that the first species cannot produce itself.

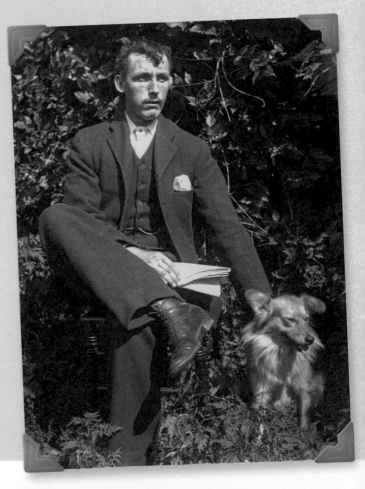

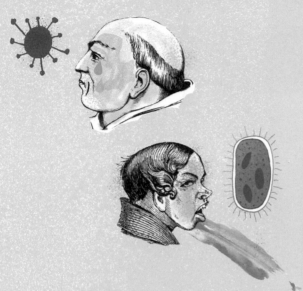

Not all parasites are pathogens, just those that cause disease in humans.

COMMENSALISM

A symbiotic relationship that is neither beneficial nor harmful to either species. Often one species may obtain shelter or transport from the other, without causing any noticeable harm. Many of the body's microbes are commensal.

PARASITISM

A symbiotic relationship in which one species (the parasite) lives on or in another (the host) and causes harm, weakening the host or worse. A pathogen is a parasite that specifically causes disease in humans, and the term is often reserved for microbes. An organism may be parasitic, but not necessarily pathogenic. Intestinal worms, for example, can steal nutrients from you, but do not necessarily cause disease.

The symbiotic relationship with opportunistic pathogens (see pages 18–19) shifts from commensalism to pathogenic.

COMMUNICATION IS KEY

Good communication is key to any long-lasting relationship. Despite being very different organisms, your cells use many of the same compounds for communication as bacterial cells. Scientists estimate that 37 percent of human genes are related to bacteria genes, and most of the proteins these genes make are important for communication between bacteria and animals.

If you consider that commensal bacteria have probably been exchanging information throughout the seven million years of human evolution (if you include the earliest human-like ancestors), it is plausible to think that this relationship has shaped the evolution of each of the organisms involved — as scientists now believe.

LONG-TERM RELATIONSHIPS

Organisms in long-term symbiotic relationships (symbionts) co-evolve with each other. Some scientists think that gut bacteria have shaped the evolution of mammalian guts, particularly ruminants (grazing animals such as cattle), enabling food to pass through the gut more slowly and so give bacteria longer access to the nutrients. Another theory suggests that bacteria may have played a role in the evolution of warm-blooded animals (endothermy). Human body temperature (98.6°F/37°C) happens also to be the optimal temperature for our symbiotic bacteria. The more scientists learn about our good bacteria, the more they believe that these have actively shaped their environment in their favor.

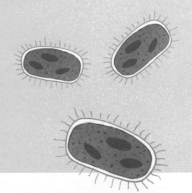

A DAY IN THE LIFE OF BACTERIA

At first glance, a bacterium's diary might seem rather boring — eat and divide, eat and divide. However, bacteria have to pack a lot of activities into their "day." These help them not only to survive, but also to improve their current environment and prepare for any changes in the future.

Just as your "to do" list probably includes jobs associated with work, home, health, family life and leisure, the tasks of a bacterium can be loosely categorized in the same way.

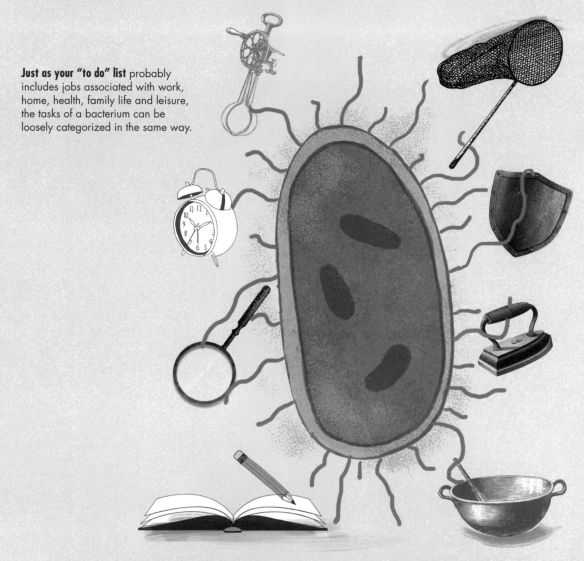

WORK

While bacteria certainly aren't putting in a 60-hour week to get ahead in the workplace, they do perform tasks that enable them to acquire more resources. *Lactobacillus* in your gut, for example, spends a good portion of its time converting sugars into lactate (lactic acid) and, much to your benefit, manufacturing Vitamin K through fermentation in order to get energy. Bacteria need energy to perform all the other tasks required to grow and reproduce. If you eat at regular times, *Lactobacillus* will respond to your daily agenda and begin to divide rapidly in anticipation of receiving more "work" to do — essentially developing a team of worker clones.

HOME

Just as we like to make our homes more pleasant to live in, so bacteria monitor and make improvements to their habitat. They communicate both with their co-habiting bacteria and with the host itself in order to keep the household as stable as possible. *Lactobacillus* produces hydrogen peroxide (H_2O_2), which keeps its environment free of the nutrient-stealing *Candida albicans*, for example.

PERSONAL WELL-BEING

Bacteria have to spend time maintaining their cells. Activities include removing waste from the cell, repairing DNA and building proteins and other molecules that the cell will use once it is ready to divide. Bacteria also come under attack from viruses (bacteriophages), so personal tasks might include destroying the DNA of an invading virus.

A BACTERIUM'S "DAY" CAN BE VERY SHORT. THE AVERAGE LIFE OF A SINGLE CELL OF PSEUDOMONAS NATRIEGENS, AN OCEAN-DWELLING BACTERIUM, IS 10 MINUTES. THIS IS THE TIME FROM WHEN A NEW CELL FORMS TO WHEN IT DIVIDES AGAIN.

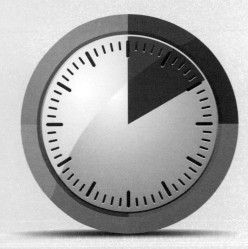

FAMILY

The ultimate goal of a bacterium is to replicate its DNA and physically divide. As an individual cell it is limited in what it can accomplish, but thousands, if not millions, of cells will contain enough genetic diversity (see pages 28–29) to let some individuals adapt to new situations, allowing their genes to live on. With division a priority, it is not surprising that much of what a bacterium does relates to achieving this primary task. For example, *E. coli* spends approximately 45 percent of the time between forming a new cell and dividing again in making a copy of its genome; another 33 percent is spent physically dividing the cell. Taken together, that's more than 75 percent of the bacterium's lifetime!

BACTERIA MOVE IN

You come in contact with bacteria every day. Most of these bacteria end up passing through — quite literally, in the case of your gut — because they cannot survive in the habitats your body provides. Some bacteria, however, quite happily take up residence.

THE PERFECT HOME

Many aspects of the human body make it an ideal environment for certain species of microbe.

WARMTH: All the bacteria associated with humans, good and bad, tend to find temperatures between 86°F and 104°F (30°C–40°C) ideal — so the human body's 98.6°F (37°C) is perfect.

MOISTURE: Bacteria are largely composed of water, which is essential for them to carry out reactions in the cell, dissolve nutrients and grow. This is why there are a plethora of bacteria around all your body's sweaty spots (e.g. armpits) and mucous membranes (e.g. nose).

You acquire bacteria from three main sources: from your mother at birth, from the food you eat and from your environment.

Propionibacterium acnes lives on the skin but does not like oxygen, so it lives deep inside the skin's hair follicles, feeding on the oils produced by skin glands.

present, such as as your skin, while your intestine is filled largely with anaerobic bacteria.

SPACE: Bacteria generally grow better when attached to surfaces, so physical space can also be an important factor for thriving microbes.

Environments in which bacteria cannot survive are usually just extreme versions of the conditions that they like. It is by creating these extreme conditions that food is preserved, in order to prevent bacteria from growing and spoiling it. For example, all the moisture is removed from meat to make jerky, chicken is cooked to kill *Campylobacter*, *Staphylococcus* and other bad bacteria, and pickling lowers the pH so that bad bacteria cannot grow.

MAKING MINOR RENOVATIONS

When some microbes take up residence they can begin to alter their environment slightly in order to make it more suitable. For example, a common bacterium that lives on your skin, *Propionibacterium acnes*, breaks down the fat-rich substance that glands in the skin produce to lubricate and protect your hair and skin; this releases free fatty acids that help the bacterium stick to the skin. Incidentally, it also makes the skin slightly more acidic, which inhibits the growth of bad bacteria such as *Streptococcus pyogenes*, a cause of impetigo and other skin infections.

PH: The acidity or alkalinity of an environment affects how well the enzymes necessary for cellular reactions work. While most of your body is a relatively neutral pH, your gut most certainly is not. The gut bacteria, such as those belonging to the groups *Bifidobacterium* and *Lactobacillus*, have found different ways to keep their internal pH neutral while living in this hostile acid environment.

NUTRIENTS: Bacteria, like all living things, need nutrients to survive. For gut bacteria, this is generally fiber, and for those living on your skin it might be dead skin cells.

OXYGEN (OR NOT): Some species of bacteria require oxygen (aerobic). Others find it poisonous (anaerobic) and yet others, such as *Escherichia coli*, can live in either condition (facultative anaerobe). Aerobic bacteria can only live where oxygen is

YOUR MICROBE MAP

Species of bacteria thrive in different areas of your body depending on the environment. The microbial communities associated with your skin, oral cavity and gut are as dissimilar as the animals native to Australia, North America and Antarctica. In fact, the microbes on an Australian coral reef are more similar to those found on a Canadian prairie than the microbes living in your mouth are to those living not far away in your gut.

Different parts of your body not only vary in which species of bacteria are present, but also in the number of species (richness) and the abundance of each of those species. Your skin, for example, has a larger number of species present, but your gut contains a far greater quantity of microbes in total (just fewer species). This is mainly because your skin comes into contact with far more bacteria through your environment, while only limited numbers of species are capable of coping with the acidic environment of the gut.

Some of these communities also change more frequently than others. Our hands, for example, might be exposed to more bacteria because we do so much with them, but they are also washed more frequently. Compare that with the moist area between the toes or the crease at the back of the knees: here microbe communities are more stable because they are not disturbed as often.

GATHERING AROUND RESOURCES

Microbes are distributed around the body much as people are in the landscape, with densely populated "urban" areas and more sparsely populated "rural" areas.

Microbes gather around resources, just as towns might develop around a particular industry. On the skin, hair follicles and sweat pores provide a veritable geyser of salts, vitamins, amino acids and sugars for bacteria. As a result, the highest densities of bacteria can be found here.

A UNIQUE MAP

Although you might only share 10 percent of the same species of microbes as a stranger on the street, the areas where microbes particularly like to gather — feet, gut and so on — are similar for everyone. But some things you do can affect the location of the "urban centers" on your microbe map. If you wear spectacles, for example, you are likely to have a very unique community of bacteria on the bridge of your nose, where your glasses rest. Women typically have a "necklace" of bacteria where their application of face cream ends. Skin products, jewellery and the material of your clothing (natural or synthetic) can also all influence your unique microbe map.

Many bacteria appear very similar through a microscope. In order to look at the different microbial communities living with us, scientists sequence the bacterial DNA, building a map of microbes based on their genome.

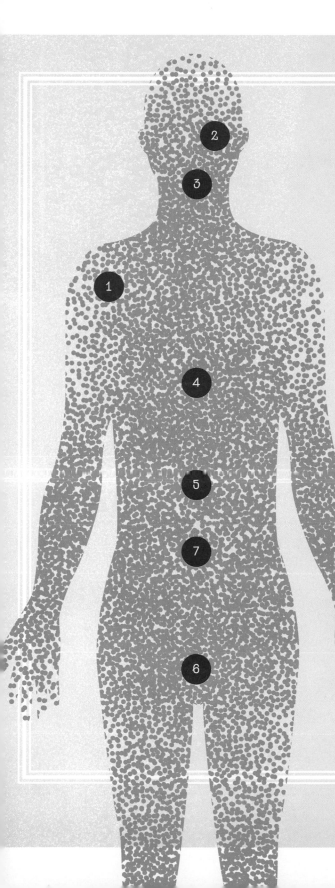

MAPPING THE MICROBIOME

Bacteria live in and on most of the body, but play a significant role in the areas highlighted here: we focus on these in Chapter 2.

1. SKIN
2. EYES
3. MOUTH
4. LUNGS
5. GUT
6. UROGENITAL SYSTEM
7. WOMB (PREGNANCY AND NEWBORN BABY)

BREVIBACTERIUM LINENS FOUND ON THE SKIN CREATES SMELLY ODORS ON THE FEET. IT IS ALSO USED TO MAKE SOME CHEESES, HENCE THEIR "SWEATY SOCK" SMELL

DIVISION AND DIVERSITY

Bacteria, like all living creatures, have a primal urge to pass on their DNA, but they do not even need a mate. Bacteria reproduce through a process known as fission, in which a single cell divides to become two smaller daughter cells. These contain exactly the same DNA as the parent cell.

When a bacterium is ready to divide all the DNA, including any non-chromosomal DNA (plasmids) that the cell contains, is duplicated. Each daughter cell has one strand of the original parental DNA, along with a new complementary strand built up using proteins and amino acids from within the cell.

A bacterium needs to be large enough to contain at least two copies of its DNA (black and blue circular scribbles) before it can begin to divide.

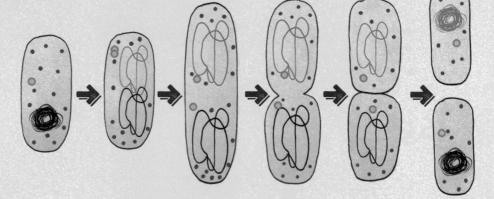

DOUBLING TIME

The time that it takes for bacteria to go through fission depends on many things, including their species, environment and the nutrients available. When most individuals in a population of bacteria (see page 11) have undergone fission, the population size doubles. This rate of growth, known as doubling or generation time, is an important measure in bacteriology, as it is an indicator of how quickly a species can expand and spread.

While being able to split into two makes the dating scene much easier in the bacterial world, it does not introduce a lot of diversity. Genetic clones all share the same DNA, and so have all the same strengths and weaknesses when it comes to responding to changes in their environment.

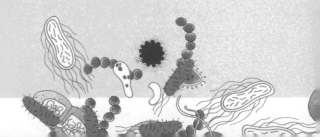

INTRODUCING SOME DIVERSITY

Genetic diversity gives all living organisms a better chance of adapting to and surviving changes in their environment. Bacteria have a number of ways of acquiring new genetic material, which may (or may not) contain helpful genes that improve their success.

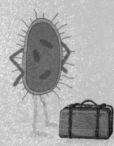

TRANSFORMATION
A bacterium might encounter strands of loose DNA in its environment, which it can absorb through the cell membrane.

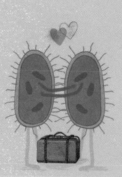

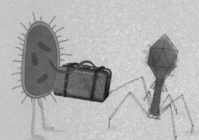

TRANSDUCTION
Viruses that prey on bacteria often contain DNA from their previous host. When the virus infects a new bacterium, it injects that bacterial DNA into its new host.

CONJUGATION
The closest thing to sex in the bacterial world. One bacterium (the donor) uses a hair-like appendage called a pilus to pull another nearby bacterium (the recipient) toward it. When the two bacteria are touching, any plasmid DNA is replicated and a copy given to the recipient. The recipient has now acquired the ability to form a pilus and donate to other cells in turn.

PUTTING NEW DNA TO USE
Picking up sections of new DNA is one thing, but the bacterium needs to incorporate these into its existing DNA to make use of them. The new DNA can either be incorporated into the bacterium's chromosomal DNA or it can form its own plasmid. It will then pass on this revised genome to its clone daughter cells when it divides. The genes on this DNA may be of no use at all, or they may give the bacterium an advantage in, say, warmer temperatures, or provide it with resistance against certain antibiotics. It is this transfer of DNA and their speedy generation time that help bacteria to evolve rapidly and spread particularly useful genes, such as antibiotic resistance, very quickly through a population.

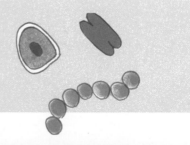

MUTATIONS AND THEIR CONSEQUENCES

Just like any other living cell, bacteria are prone to the occasional spontaneous genetic change, known as a mutation. An organism's genetic code is often likened to a recipe book, from which cells choose recipes for specific proteins as needed. Mutations can cause an ingredient to be substituted or even an entire recipe to be altered or lost, sometimes with serious consequences.

If DNA is the recipe book, then a gene is equivalent to a recipe. Escherichia coli's own "recipe book" contains about 5,000 recipes, each providing the instructions to make a protein.

ESCHERICHIA COLI'S TOP 5,000 RECIPES

INGREDIENTS

THE BOOK OF DNA

METHOD

1. MUTATIONS IN THE GENETIC CODE ARE RELATIVELY RARE EVENTS. THEY MAY GO COMPLETELY UNNOTICED, AS IF YOU HAD SWAPPED SKIM MILK IN A PANCAKE RECIPE.

2. SOMETIMES, HOWEVER, THE MUTATION MIGHT BE DETRIMENTAL TO THE BACTERIUM — PERHAPS IT CANNOT PRODUCE AN ENZYME IT NEEDS, OR ITS GROWTH IS SOMEHOW SLOWED.

3. A BACTERIUM WITH A DETRIMENTAL MUTATION WILL EITHER CEASE TO BE VIABLE OR WILL BE OUTCOMPETED BY ITS NON-MUTATED CLONE COMPANIONS. EITHER WAY, THE MUTATION GETS "SELECTED OUT" OF THE BACTERIA POPULATION.

POWERFUL MUTANTS

Occasionally, however, a mutation might be advantageous. For example, the mutation might make a bacterium faster at DNA replication, or provide it with resistance to certain viruses. The beneficial mutation is passed on to the daughter cells, allowing them in turn to outcompete non-mutant cells, generating more clones with the mutation. Eventually, the beneficial mutation becomes dominant in the bacteria population.

MUTATION RATES

Spontaneous mutations are relatively rare. As a bacterium makes repairs to its DNA before it replicates, many of these events are in fact caught by the cell's quality control. However, the speedy division time of bacteria means that even these rare mutation events can build up over a short period of time, leading to numerous mutants in a population. In just 10 hours, for example, a single *Staphylococcus aureus* cell can lead to a colony of one million cells with nearly 300 mutants.

Mutations happen spontaneously, but certain factors increase the chances of their occurrence. These include free radicals (highly reactive molecules produced through normal chemical reactions in the cell), ultraviolet radiation from the sun and chemicals such as antibiotics.

When bacteria are stressed, genes kick into gear that essentially shut down the cell's quality control department (or at least leave it understaffed). The resulting higher mutation rate increases the chances of a mutation that might help the bacteria, such as the ability to make use of a new nutrient. If the environment is stable, however, it is too risky to have a high mutation rate as there is more chance of producing harmful mutations than beneficial ones. In such conditions it is better to stick with the recipes that work.

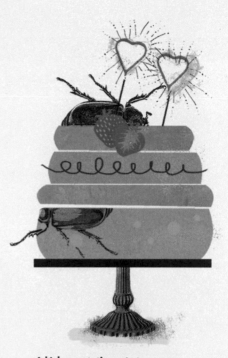

A higher mutation rate increases the likelihood that a population of bacteria will find that show-stopping recipe that enables some of them to survive in a stressful situation. However, the vast majority of mutations will not be useful to the bacteria at all.

THE BAD BACTERIA IN YOUR MICROBIOME TEND TO HAVE HIGHER MUTATION RATES THAN THE GOOD BACTERIA. THIS IS PROBABLY BECAUSE THEY ARE FREQUENTLY UNDER ATTACK BY YOUR BODY'S IMMUNE SYSTEM. UNFORTUNATELY, THIS MEANS THAT THE BACTERIA WE MOST WANT TO GET RID OF ARE THOSE MOST LIKELY TO ADAPT TO MEDICINES SUCH AS ANTIBIOTICS.

THE INFECTION PROCESS

Just as good bacteria need to find a suitable place to live in and on your body, so do bad bacteria. Without this they cannot grow and multiply. Unlike good bacteria, however, bad bacteria have to do battle with all your good microbes as well as your immune system as they try to colonize your body. Most fail, but some do manage to get through your body's defenses.

INFECTION STARTS

Infection might begin with a sneeze or a hand-shake, maybe a contaminated kitchen counter or a dubious burger. Perhaps you cut yourself, compro-mising your body's first line of defense — your skin. There might be a "middle-man," or vector, such as a tick or mosquito that bites you, injecting microbe-filled saliva into your bloodstream. There are many direct and indirect pathways through which you come into contact with bad bacteria. Your body is incredibly good at defending itself (see pages 34–37), but these bad bacteria have evolved an ar-senal of weapons to help them colonize, reproduce and spread.

INVADING THE HOST

Any invading force requires strength in numbers, and bacteria are no different. The more bacteria there are infiltrating your tissues, the greater the chance that they will be able to overwhelm your immune system. Each species of bad bacteria requires a different number of cells in order to have an effect — known as the infectious dose.

Streptococcus suis can cause meningitis, septicaemia and other serious diseases in humans. It is one of many species of bacteria to release a toxin that quite literally drills holes in the walls of animal cells, so killing them.

Shigella dysenteriae, for example, only requires 10–200 cells to take hold and start causing dysentery. *Campylobacter jejuni*, on the other hand — a common source of food poisoning associated with chicken — requires at least 10,000 cells to cause illness because the majority will not survive the hostile acidic conditions of your gut. Some bacteria are so virulent that fewer than 10 cells can cause an infection, possibly even a single cell (though this is not yet known for sure). These include *Escherichia coli* O157:H7 and *Mycobacterium tuberculosis*.

CAUSING DISEASE

Bad bacteria may infect your tissues, but not actually cause disease. In other words, they manage to colonize your tissues (infection), without causing any symptoms of illness. This is known as a subclinical infection. However, in many other cases, an infection can lead to disease. This happens in one of two ways. Bad bacteria may crowd out the host tissues, disrupting them in a way that prevents them from working properly, much as a tumor does. Alternatively, the bacteria might kill your body's cells outright using toxins.

Bad bacteria infect your tissues when the balance between their virulence and your resistance tip in the bacteria's favor. A bacteria's virulence is measured by its ability to invade the host, evade defenses and then cause disease once it is established there.

IN A SINGLE SNEEZE THERE CAN BE AS MANY AS 40,000 DROPLETS OF WATER, ALL CARRYING BACTERIA

THE IMMUNE SYSTEM

When your cells detect bad bacteria, they sound an alarm to call in the troops. This uses chemicals that kick the immune cells in the local area into action (the front line). If they cannot beat the infection, the heavy artillery are summoned.

Innate vs adaptive: the immune system has a non-specific defense system that responds rapidly to any foreign invader — known as innate immunity. This is in addition to a set of cells that respond specifically to invaders they have encountered before, known as adaptive immunity.

THE FRONT LINE

Granulocytes, macrophages, NK (natural killer) cells and mast cells are the first immune cells to react to an infection. Granulocytes and macrophages immediately start to engulf or "eat" the bacteria and break them down. These immune cells then display parts of the bacteria on their cell surface, showing other immune cells what to look for. Granulocytes also release chemicals that break down the bacterial cell wall. NK cells attack human cells infected by the bacteria. Mast cells send out chemicals known as histamines. These alert immune cells in other parts of the body so that they can come and join in the attack.

THE HEAVY ARTILLERY

If the infection cannot be controlled quickly, the heavy artillery is required. Specialized cells, known as B cells, start producing antibodies that bind to the intruding bacteria, making it easier for the other cells of the immune system to recognize and destroy them. The antibodies can also help to stick the bacteria together, so that large groups of them can be engulfed at once. Other specialized cells, known as T cells, assist by attacking infected cells and stimulating B cells to produce more antibodies. The B cells and T cells also keep a record of the attack, enabling your immune system to react even faster if you encounter those bacteria again.

BACTERIA FIGHT BACK

Bacteria have evolved a number of defense strategies against the immune system. They can disguise themselves to try and evade detection. For example, *Streptococcus pneumoniae* (which causes pneumonia) constantly changes the proteins it puts on its cell surface in the hope that the immune system won't recognize it; scientists have identified 84 different "uniforms" that the invading *S. pneumoniae* wears. Some species of bacteria suppress the immune system, slowing down the activity of the immune cells. *Streptococcus pyogenes* produces an enzyme that slows and weakens immune cells.

A number of species of bacteria use interference strategies in their fight back against the immune system. *Haemophilus influenzae* (causes infections, but not influenza, which is viral) releases chemicals that break down antibodies and *S. aureus* ejects protein molecules out from its cell wall. Antibodies bind to these molecules mistaking them for the bacteria. Once bound, the antibodies are useless. Other bacteria hide from the immune system. *Listeria* (causes food poisoning) hides within the immune cells that have engulfed it but manages to avoid being destroyed, while *Streptococcus mutans* (causes tooth decay) hangs out on your teeth, where scientists believe the immune cells cannot reach it.

SYMPTOMS OF AN IMMUNE REACTION

The symptoms associated with an infection — fever, headache and inflammation — are actually the result of your immune system's response to the infection rather than the infection itself. The release of histamines, as anyone who suffers from hay fever will know, not only calls in the heavy artillery, but also triggers a number of responses from other cells. Cells that line your sinuses, for example, start to produce more mucus as a further barrier to the invading bacteria. You feel tired. Your body begins to shiver and rise in temperature, causing fever, and you may get a headache. Blood vessels dilate so that cells of the immune system can travel more easily, but this also causes redness and inflammation. Many of the uncomfortable symptoms of an infection are in fact the body's immune system responding to attack.

SEPSIS

When the body's immune response is too strong it begins to affect the normal functioning of your cells. It may cause dangerously high fever, rapid breathing and abnormal heart beat — a reaction known as sepsis or blood poisoning. The infection itself is known as septicaemia. When the immune system overreacts to this infection, it is a serious complication, as inflammation in the region of the infection starts to spread to healthy tissues. Sepsis is rare, but unless treated quickly it can lead to multiple organ failure and even death.

HOMEOSTASIS

We have discussed how the immune system responds to alarm calls within the body. However, there is also a constant chemical chatter between your cells, letting all the systems know they are working well, to which the immune system also responds. This is known as homeostasis — a balance between all the systems. Your microbiome is part of this regular chatter, communicating with the body through various pathways to confirm that all is well. This communication is thought to be a large part of why the body's immune system recognizes its beneficial bacteria as allies — they are just there all the time, chattering away and not causing any harm.

Macrophages extend pseudopods (arm-like extensions) when they detect bacteria, reaching out to grab the bacteria and bring them in to engulf them within the macrophage cell, where they break the bacteria down.

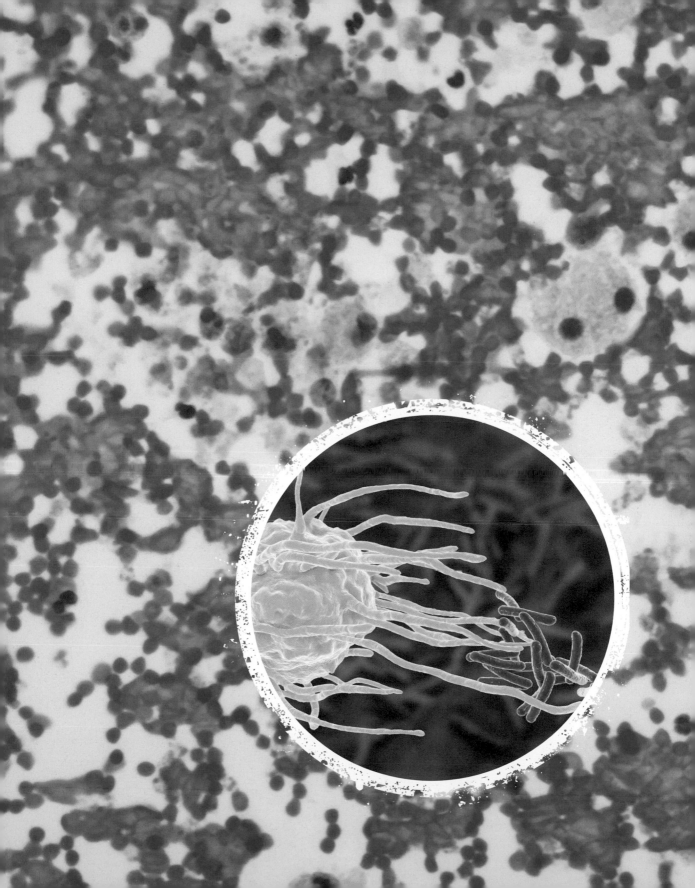

TEACHING THE IMMUNE SYSTEM

There is no database of bad guys when it comes to teaching your immune system. Your body needs to be ready to take on any foreign invader without having prior knowledge of what it is or how it operates. Your beneficial bacteria must therefore make sure that your immune system views them as one of its own — one of the good guys.

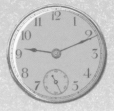

Every cell in your body displays a set of proteins on its surface, known as self-proteins, which are unique to you. Your immune cells use these proteins to help them distinguish cells that belong to you ("self") from other cells, including harmful bacteria ("non-self").

All cells have proteins embedded on their cell surface, which are known as receptors. These receptors recognize and bind to different molecules in the environment, including other cells. As immune cells develop, they shuffle proteins haphazardly to create new cell surface receptors. This is an extremely effective way of generating a battery of receptors that might one day help your immune cells recognize a foreign cell, like having a workshop stocked with tools without yet knowing what it is you have to fix. The problem with this is that because these receptors are randomly generated, there is a chance that some might recognize and bind to the "self" proteins on your cells, causing your immune cells to launch an attack on your own cells. To avoid this, each of your body's immune cells undergoes rigorous testing to ensure that it does not bind to "self" proteins. Only cells that pass these tests are permitted to "mature" and enter the body. If a cell fails the test, it is destroyed.

Your beneficial bacteria do not carry "self" proteins on their surface, so they must train the immune system to recognize them and not attack them. This training is thought to begin the moment you are born, and possibly even before.

MOTHER'S MILK

Scientists think that the live bacteria, antibodies and some other chemical compounds found in a mother's milk may help to train a baby's immune system, but they are not sure how. They have found specialized immune cells in the milk that are pre-loaded with bacteria, and suspect that these may play a role in teaching the baby's immune system how to respond to friendly bacteria.

A CALMING EFFECT

The immune system in infants is also less reactive than a mature immune system. Not having yet been exposed to the world, it has no memory of previous illnesses. This immature immune system allows bacteria to become established, with the immune system and the microbiome essentially maturing and developing together. Scientists believe that anti-inflammatory chemicals produced by the first colonizing bacteria and specialized cells in the gut "calm" the infant's immune system. If the immune system were to react to everything as it developed, it might miss the really bad bacteria amidst all the commotion.

THE PRICE OF HAVING A LESS REACTIVE IMMUNE SYSTEM IS THAT INFANTS ARE UNFORTUNATELY MORE PRONE TO INFECTIONS

ALLERGIES AND AUTOIMMUNE DISORDERS

If your immune system perceives perfectly harmless proteins in your body as being bad, it will launch an unwarranted attack. When immune cells attack proteins that are harmless to most people, such as peanut proteins, this is known as an allergy. If immune cells attack your own cells, this leads to autoimmune disease. While both allergies and autoimmune diseases are thought to be affected by your genetics and the environment, your bacteria may also have a role to play.

Allergies and autoimmune disorders are the result of an over-reactive immune system attacking harmless proteins. However, if the immune system isn't active enough (weakened or suppressed) it doesn't work properly either. It has to be just right.

OVER-REACTIVE   UNDER-REACTIVE   JUST RIGHT

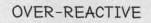

WHAT ABOUT THE PERMANENT RESIDENTS?

Research has revealed clear links between bacteria, allergies and autoimmune disease, but the detail of how these work is still being studied. Exposure to bacteria during the development of the immune system is one of many factors that might make a person more prone to allergies, asthma and/or autoimmune diseases. Yet it is still not clear what role your good bacteria play in the development (or prevention) of these conditions. There also seems to be a relationship between the amount of antibiotics a child receives in their first two years of life and their likelihood of developing allergies, suggesting that more antibiotics means an increased chance of allergies. People with allergies tend to have a different composition of bacteria in their guts — often having a lower proportion of beneficial bacteria from the groups *Bacteroides* and *Lactobacilli*.

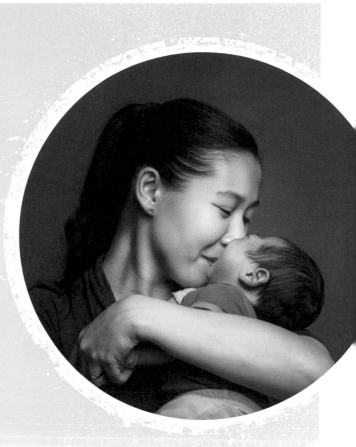

RESTORING BALANCE

While scientists try and resolve different pieces of the puzzle, the common finding is that your good bacteria seem to maintain balance in your immune system. So, just as yin and yang are opposite and yet complementary, your immune system has inflammatory and regulatory cells. Some immune cells release cytokines that create inflammation (the party-goers), while others have a regulatory effect that help maintain tolerance (the teetotallers). The presence of good bacteria in your gut seems to stimulate immature immune cells to develop into teetotallers rather than party-goers. This promotes a more tolerant immune system, less prone to unwarranted attacks.

CHILDREN BORN BY CESAREAN SECTION ARE TWICE AS LIKELY TO HAVE AN ALLERGY TO EGG OR MILK PROTEINS. THIS MAY BE A RESULT OF THE MICROBES TO WHICH THEY WERE (OR WERE NOT) EXPOSED AT BIRTH. IN THE LAST 50 YEARS, THE PROPORTION OF PEOPLE WITH ALLERGIES, ASTHMA AND AUTOIMMUNE DISEASES HAS STEADILY INCREASED. THERE IS CONSIDERABLE DEBATE ABOUT WHY THIS SHOULD BE SO. ONE OF THE PREVALENT THEORIES IS BASED ON THE FACT THAT OUR RELATIONSHIP TO BACTERIA HAS DRASTICALLY CHANGED OVER THIS PERIOD.

BACTERIA THROUGH THE AGES

You start to acquire bacteria from the moment you are born, and possibly even while still in the womb. Within three years children will develop a stable community of good bacteria. As you grow, life events such as puberty, pregnancy and illness can cause changes in this bacterial community, even if only temporarily. The microbiome then starts to shift again when you reach later life and beyond.

A STABLE COMMUNITY

The microbiome of a healthy adult is fairly stable — so much so that if you live with someone for days, weeks or even years, your microbiome may change little, despite being exposed to new species of bacteria through the relationship. A stable community of bacteria can resist minor disturbances, such as illness or a bout of antibiotics, over the short to medium term. Your microbiome resembles a well-established, old-growth forest in which the species composition remains quite constant. However, much like a mature forest, it takes a little while for the community of bacteria to establish itself.

NEWBORN

How and where a baby enters the world directly affects the species of bacteria with which he or she first comes into contact (see pages 132–33). The bacteria may be from the vagina or the skin, depending on whether it is a natural or cesarean birth, for instance. If babies are born in unhygienic conditions, this also influences which species of bacteria first colonize them. Babies born in Sub-Saharan Africa, for example, are 30 times more likely to get an infection within their first month of life compared with babies born in developed countries.

A baby's bacterial community is rapidly changing, but it is not particularly diverse because the baby's initial milk diet is not diverse. A baby's gut contains a large number of bacteria that produce folic acid (Vitamin B9) from the milk, which is vital for healthy infant development.

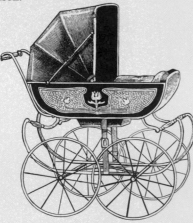

As a child grows from infant to toddler, the development of its microbiome is similar to the way in which plants and animals colonize a newly formed island, eventually growing into a diverse ecosystem.

TODDLERS AND ONWARD

Toddlers are more mobile and inquisitive than babies, and as a result are exposed to far more bacteria, the types of which depend on where they live (see pages 166–67). As they grow, their microbial community starts to become more diverse. Toddlers also eat a more diverse range of food, from which they receive most of their micronutrients. Unlike infants, toddlers get most of their folic acid from their food, so the species of bacteria in their gut change to folic acid harvesters, efficient at collecting folic acid from food.

Before the age of three, there is more variation in one child's gut bacteria from week to week than there is between two healthy adults — which is in itself substantial. As a child's gut bacteria start to resemble the same types as in an adult's gut, the community starts to stabilize.

CHILDHOOD

The microbiome of children experiences minor fluctuations during bouts of illness, but otherwise remains stable until changes in the gut start to occur with old age.

After the age of three, a child's microbiome begins to settle down into the one it will take into adulthood, hence the need to encourage a healthy microbiome from very early childhood.

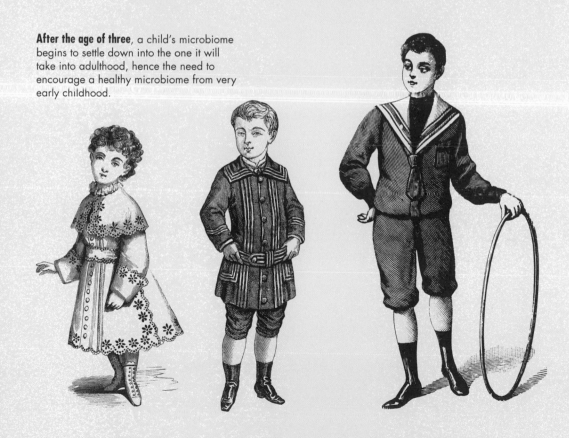

PUBERTY

The skin bacteria are affected when the hormone surges experienced by preteens and teens at the onset of puberty stimulate the skin's sebaceous glands to produce copious amounts of a waxy substance known as sebum. This lubricates the skin, and provides more resources for *Propionibacterium acnes* — the most common species associated with skin (see page 65).

ADULTHOOD

The microbiome of an adult is well-established and remains relatively stable. Lifestyle factors, such as diet, sleep cycles and exercise affect the microbiome (see pages 156–57), as does illness. Major life events can also have an impact. A woman, for example, will experience a change in the bacteria that inhabit her vagina if she becomes pregnant.

Certain species become more common, and these will ultimately be the bacteria that help to colonize the newborn infant.

GETTING OLDER

As a person ages, further changes occur. The body's cells do not regenerate as easily, hormones change, hair becomes thinner, food is digested more slowly and the body's activity level may drop, altering the habitats in which its friendly bacteria live. For example older skin is dryer, thinner and less elastic, while the density of pores decreases. As a result, the *Propionibacterium* species reduce, making room for other species to colonize. It is not yet known whether losing the *Propionibacterium* group may actually contribute to the signs of skin aging. Perhaps future anti-wrinkle creams will contain a dose of beneficial bacteria?

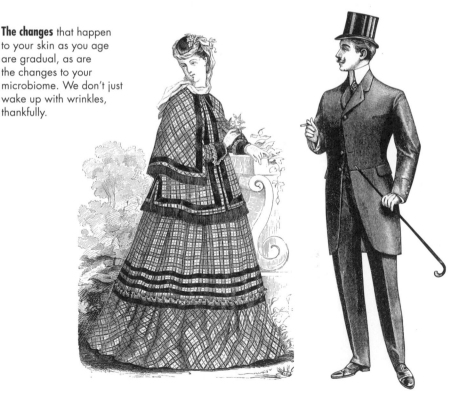

The changes that happen to your skin as you age are gradual, as are the changes to your microbiome. We don't just wake up with wrinkles, thankfully.

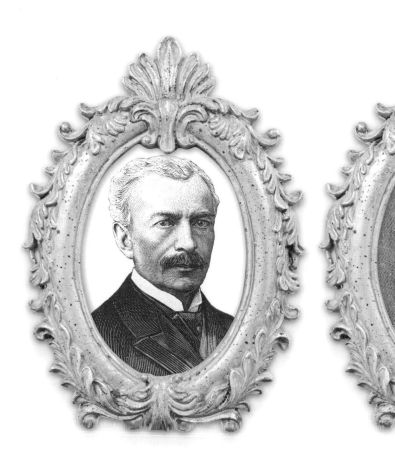

The gut environment also changes in an older person. Digestion slows down and people's food preferences can change if certain foods become hard to chew, resulting in a shift in diet. With the change in environment comes a change in the gut bacteria. *E. coli*, for example, becomes more prominent, while highly beneficial species belonging to the *Bacteroides* and *Bifidobacteria* groups are less prominent. Scientific studies are exploring how such a shift in gut bacterial species among the elderly may be related to the immune system becoming less tolerant as people age. This chronic state of inflammation in the immune system causes many of the discomforts associated with aging — known as inflammaging.

PEOPLE OVER 65 GENERALLY HAVE FEWER BACTERIAL SPECIES (NOT NECESSARILY FEWER BACTERIA).

ANTIBIOTICS

People were using antibiotics to kill bacteria long before scientists coined the term antibiotic (from "anti-," meaning against, and the Greek word "–bios," meaning life) and long before the first microscope allowed us to see bacteria.

An antibiotic is any substance that slows or stops the growth of bacteria. These substances are produced by all sorts of organisms, from other microbes through to panda bears (see pages 174–75), to defend themselves from harmful bacteria. As humans are not particularly good at producing antibiotics naturally, scientists have been identifying and isolating these substances, found throughout nature, in order to develop medicines that can help us fight bad bacteria.

HOW ANTIBIOTICS WORK

Antibiotics work by disrupting the growth of bacteria without affecting the body's own cells. They target cellular processes or parts that are unique to bacteria. Penicillin, for example, prevents bacteria from building their cell wall properly, causing them to explode when they try and divide; animal cells, including those of humans, do not have cell walls so it does not affect them.

TAKING A COURSE OF ANTIBIOTICS

Sometimes a bacterial infection is too tough for the body to fight on its own, so a health professional prescribes a course of antibiotics. The antibiotic prescribed will be as specific as possible to the bad bacteria. It will also be given for the least amount of time needed to kill them, in order to minimize damage to your good bacteria. For a urinary tract infection, for instance, you might need a three-day course, whereas sepsis might require a course of up to 10 days.

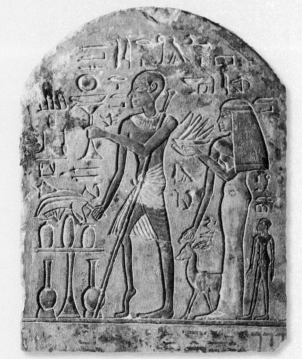

Ancient Egyptians would apply moldy bread to wounds, without realizing that it was the penicillin produced by the fungus growing on the bread that was actually helping to heal the wound.

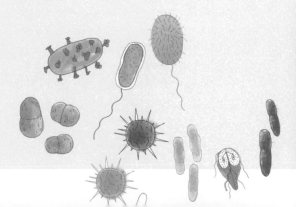

PERSISTENT BACTERIA

When you start to take antibiotics, the majority of the bad bacteria are killed off within a matter of hours. At this point you might start to feel better and may be tempted to stop the course. However, some bad bacteria will still survive because they have been less affected by the antibiotic; these are known as "persisters." If you do not finish the course, they will survive and potentially replicate, causing a second infection. This second infection might be more difficult to treat, as most of the bacteria will be descendants of the persisters and will have inherited whatever traits enabled the bacteria to hold out against the antibiotic. Some persisters have acquired genetic or physical traits through gene transfer (pages 28–29) or mutations (pages 30–31), which makes them truly resistant to the antibiotic. These are known as resistance factors. They can be transferred to other bacteria, leading to the development of super-bugs that are resistant to multiple antibiotics (pages 172–73).

Failing to finish the course of antibiotics has long been thought to increase the proportion of resistant bacteria. However, following recent research some scientists stated there was no evidence to support this. Instead they claimed that, for some bacterial infections, there might be more risk of them developing resistance if they are exposed to antibiotics for longer.

This is a complex situation in which discoveries are still to be made. For anyone prescribed antibiotics, however, the recommendation is clear: follow the advice of your health professional and if you have questions, ask.

FLEMING'S ACCIDENTAL DISCOVERY

The discovery of penicillin by Alexander Fleming, physician, biologist, pharmacologist and botanist, was quite accidental. After returning home from a brief holiday with his family in 1928, Fleming discovered that a petri plate where he had been growing *Staphylococcus* bacteria, in order to study them in greater detail, had been contaminated by a fungus. (He was well known for keeping an untidy laboratory.) None of the bacteria were growing where the fungus had grown on the plate, but, more interestingly, they were not growing even close to it. The colonies closest to the fungus were even smaller than those further away. The fungus was *Penicillium notatum*, and the antimicrobial substance that it was producing was penicillin.

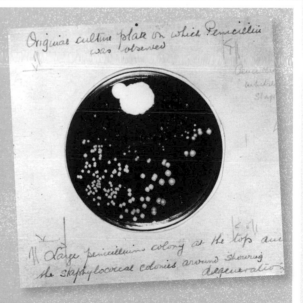

Penicillium is the large white "blob" at the top of the petri dish; the colonies of bacteria (all the small circles) closest to the fungus are much smaller.

THE HUMAN MICROBIOME PROJECT

When scientists successfully sequenced the entire human genome in 2003, it ignited an interest in sequencing another — that of our commensal microbes. There was enough evidence at this point to link human health to a healthy microbiome, but nobody had yet defined what a healthy microbiome was.

Scientists use the human microbiome reference database as a central source — just as you might use a field guide to birds to identify a common visitor to your bird feeder. Sponsored by the U.S. National Institutes of Health, the Human Microbiome Project launched in 2008. Scientists collected bacteria from 15 body locations on each of 129 men, and from 18 body locations on each of 113 women (all from the U.S.), all of whom met the strict definition of "healthy." Specimens were collected from nine areas in and around the mouth: saliva, cheek, gums, palate, tonsils, throat, tongue, and from the teeth below and above the gum line. Four skin specimens were taken: behind each ear and from the two inner elbows. A stool specimen was collected for the gut microbes, and a swab of the nostrils was taken too. Women also supplied an additional three specimens from different locations in the vagina. Eventually the scientists had 4,788 specimens to analyze.

Scientists use the human microbiome data as birdwatchers use their field guides.

THE SCIENTISTS INVOLVED IN THE HUMAN MICROBIOME PROJECT HAVE ESTIMATED THAT THERE ARE MORE THAN 10,000 DIFFERENT MICROBIAL SPECIES ASSOCIATED WITH HUMANS

A tale of two cities

If we were to list the full names of everyone living in Paris and Tokyo, very few would match. However, both cities have many accountants, athletes, chefs, cleaners, doctors and entrepreneurs.

DIVERSITY

One of the main areas the scientists looked at was diversity — the number and abundance of the different bacterial species, and whether the diversity of bacteria varied in the different areas of the body of one person. They also studied whether the diversity of bacteria collected from the same location on different people was similar. For example, did all the volunteers have the same species of bacteria living in their nostrils? The scientists found that saliva was the most diverse specimen location — the place where the greatest number of species could be found on any one person in the areas they sampled. However, many people were found to have similar bacterial species living in their saliva, so it was not as diverse between individuals. Meanwhile the bacteria living on the skin varied tremendously between people, but was of modest diversity within the same individual.

The scientists did not discover a single bacterial species that was found in or on all human habitats or associated with all individuals. The level of diversity was considerable; it made clear just how unique every individual's microbiome is to them.

The scientists also examined what the microbes did rather than what species they were. They found that everyone had roughly the same number of species that could break down carbohydrates in their gut, for example, even though the species might be quite different.

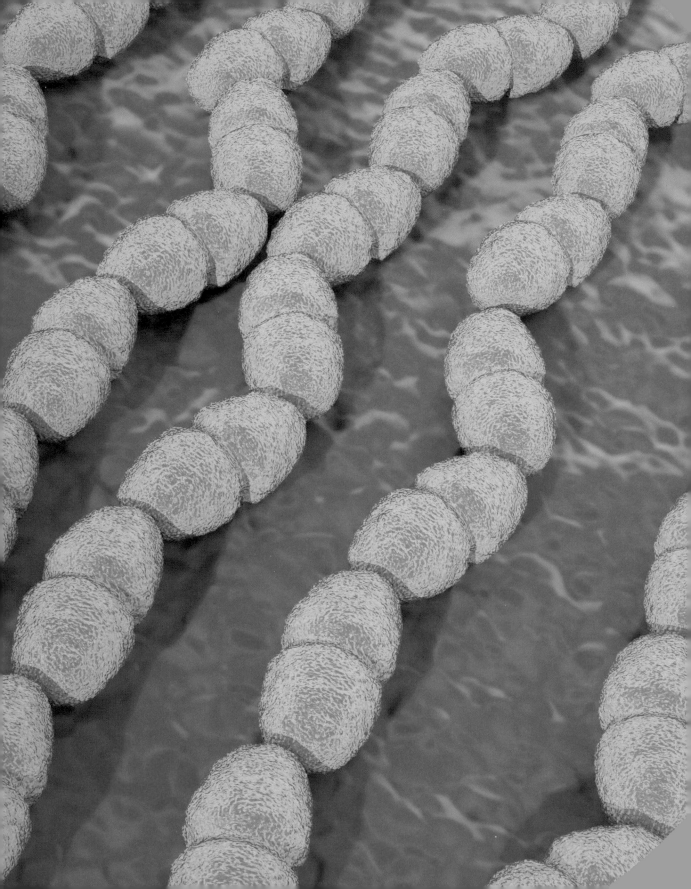

CHAPTER TWO

MAPPING THE HUMAN MICROBIOME

The contours and folds of our external and internal surfaces provide a wealth of habitats for our diverse communities of bacteria. Every human body contains as many bacteria as there are human cells, but no two people share the same bacterial profile. The location on the body determines which bacteria reside there. And while some species of bacteria are more common in one area than another, it is the jobs they perform and how they influence our lives that catch the attention.

What follows gives an insight into the bacteria that live in and on us, with advice on how to encouraage the good and discourage the bad. Every area of the body is colonized but the focus is on those areas that are constantly exposed to the world and that perform vital functions: the skin, eye, mouth, lungs, gut and urogenital system. We also look at bacteria in pregnancy and birth and how to modulate a baby's microbiome to help give an infant the best start in life.

Enterococcus fecalis bacteria

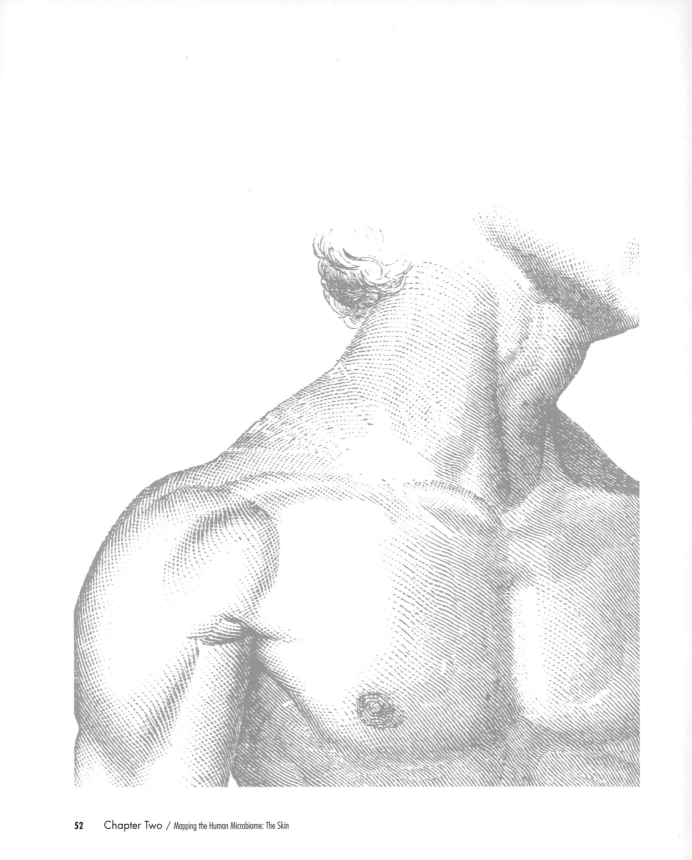

THE SKIN

The skin is the human body's largest organ. It is colonized by a diverse range of bacteria, most harmless or even beneficial to us. Some are pathogenic, but scientists now believe that the scales are weighted in favor of the good guys when it comes to skin health.

....

....

WHERE AND HOW BACTERIA LIVE ON OUR SKIN

The skin provides bacteria with a range of habitats, from the cool, dry desert of the forearm to the warm, humid jungles of the armpits or the oily sites of the face and back. Since most of the skin is exposed to the air, oxygen-loving aerobic bacteria thrive here. More hidden areas, such as sweat glands, house oxygen-hating anaerobes, for example *Propionibacterium acnes*, the bacteria involved in acne.

Thousands of different bacteria can live on the skin, so many that it is difficult to imagine how they all find space. In a study of the microbiome carried out in 2008, a total of 4,742 different species were found on 51 healthy human palms, with an average of 158 species coexisting on a single palm. The *Staphylococcus* and *Propionibacterium* species are the most common, with numerous different types of each species present on the skin.

STRUCTURE OF THE SKIN

The organs and tissues that make up the human body are too complex to expose to the outside world. The skin that encases them is composed of three layers: the epidermis, dermis and a fatty layer. Some bacteria live on the outer layer,

or epidermis, while many are associated directly or indirectly with the sweat glands in the dermis. These are concentrated in the underarms, genital area, nipples and the belly button. Hair follicles, also in the dermis, provide an attractive habitat for bacteria in the area just below the skin surface.

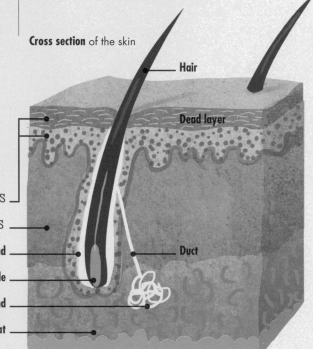

Cross section of the skin

Hair

Dead layer

EPIDERMIS

DERMIS

Sebaceous gland

Hair follicle

Sweat gland

Fat

Duct

SKIN BACTERIA

The bacteria on the skin vary according to the habitat.
They include:

OILY SITES, *such as (1) FOREHEAD, (2) BACK:*
PROPIONIBACTERIUM SPECIES, such as P. ACNES.

DRY SITES *(the most diverse), such as (3) FOREARM,*
(4) BUTTOCK: MANY SPECIES OF ACTINOBACTERIA,
PROTEOBACTERIA, FIRMICUTES, BACTEROIDETES.

MOIST SITES *such as (5) ARMPITS, GROIN, NAVEL,*
(6) SOLES OF THE FEET: STAPHYLOCOCCUS, CORYNEBACTERIUM
SPECIES, including S. EPIDERMIDIS and S. AUREUS.

PROVIDING FOR OUR BACTERIA

The surface of the skin is generally acidic, which
helps commensal bacteria, such as *Propioni-*
bacterium, adhere to the skin. The high salt concentration suits species such as *Staphylococcus*, which
have evolved to thrive in this environment.

The secretions of the skin glands are rich in nutrients for bacteria, such as urea, amino acids, salts,
lactic acid and lipids. The face and back are dominated by *Propionibacterium* species, which feed
off the fats released by the densely packed pores in
these areas. In contrast, the forearms and elbows
host a far more diverse community. The humid
areas of the navel, underarms and groin
are dominated by *Corynebacterium* species,
which feeds off the nitrogen in our sweat.

SHARING THE LOVE

We pick up bacteria on our skin from the moment of birth (see pages 132–33), and continue to change our skin bacterial profile as we go through life. Every form of contact that our body has — whether with another object or with the air — is a chance for bacteria to get on board and a single contact is enough. In Amsterdam's Micropia, the world's first museum devoted entirely to microbes, a "Kiss-o-Meter" is featured. A couple stand on a heart-shaped platform, kiss and discover how many bacteria they have just exchanged.

People who live in close contact with each other tend to harbor similar communities of bacteria. For skin bacteria a single encounter is sufficient. Students who use the same kitchen share more skin bacteria than friends who live in different houses. Contact is everything.

Shaking hands is one of the main ways bacteria are transferred from person to person. Washing hands well minimizes this method of transfer.

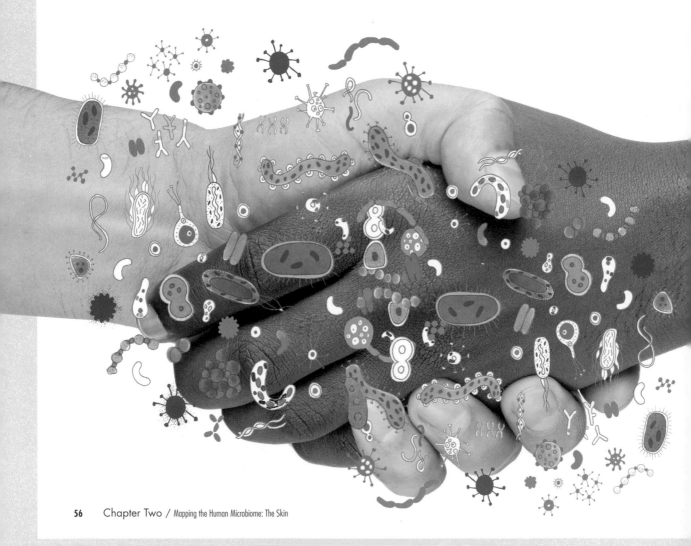

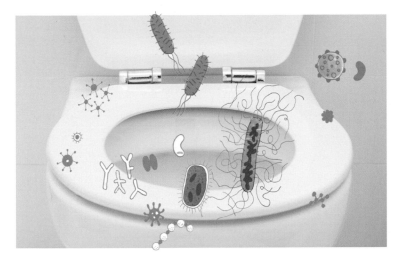

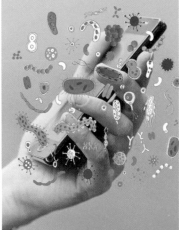

Surprisingly, toilet seats are not the dirtiest surfaces we encounter. Perhaps because they are cleaned regularly, they are less dirty than keyboards and the worst offenders — mobile phones.

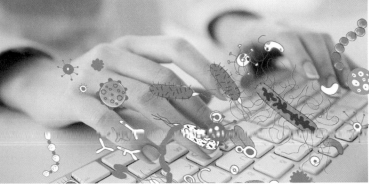

CURL UP AND DYE

A visit to the beauty parlour highlights two other popular locations for bacteria — hair and nails. These are made of keratin, a dead material, but there is a lively bacterial world on combs and nail clippers.

Hair may be dead, but its surface still supports the growth of numerous bacteria. And they get everywhere. Forensic scientists have long used hair samples as evidence in criminal cases, and the practice has now been taken one step further. A study in 2014 revealed that bacterial genetic profiling of hair could be a valuable addition to forensic science techniques.

Fingernails contain similar bacteria to the rest of the hand: just a lot more of them. The environment under the nail is perfect for bacteria. It is protected by the hard material of the nail, the keratin, and has just the right amount of moisture.

You might think twice about your next visit to the nail bar. In a study in 1989, nurses with artificial nails were shown to carry significantly more bacteria than those with unpainted nails or even painted nails. This is partly due to the length of the artificial talons, although only some of those extra bacteria will be harmful. However, it does argue that short and scrubbed nails are more hygienic.

57

BREAKING THROUGH THE SKIN LINE

The skin provides a very effective natural barrier against bacterial infection, both in the form of a physical barrier and the bacterial populations themselves, which constitute a second "skin." These bacteria simply take up space that could otherwise be invaded by pathogenic bacteria. It is estimated that only 1 percent of skin diseases are caused by bacteria, but when the skin is penetrated bacteria can cause infections, either within the skin or deeper inside the body. The predominant bacteria in skin infections are the *Staphylococcus* and *Streptococcus* species. Some of these species can be beneficial, however, such as *Staphylococcus epidermidis* (see page 66).

Bacterial infections are either introduced when there is damage to the skin — for example by a cut — or when there are other skin conditions present, such as dermatitis, eczema or psoriasis, which weaken the skin barrier. Once the skin's physical barrier is breached, the immune systems kicks in (see page 34).

Bacterial skin diseases are not usually fatal, if they are limited to the skin, but they can be highly debilitating and are extremely common. A recent study revealed that acne was one of the three skin diseases to feature in the top ten most prevalent diseases worldwide. Impetigo (*Staphylococcus aureus*) was not far behind. It causes red sores or blisters, often with a crusty yellow appearance, and usually occurs on the face. Impetigo is most common in preschool children.

Streptococci **bacteria** (opposite page)

LOCATION, LOCATION

Skin infections may just be in the skin's top layer, or epidermis, as with impetigo or acne. Or, with more serious infections such as cellulitis, the bacteria penetrate into deeper layers, for example the dermis. In very rare cases, bacteria such as *Streptococcus pyogenes* (see page 86) can rapidly penetrate and destroy the lowest layers of the skin, causing necrotizing fasciitis. This death of the body's soft tissue has resulted in terrifying tales in the media of flesh-eating bugs.

The skin can also be a window onto systemic infections (ones that affect the whole body), such as the rash of meningococcal septicaemia (blood poisoning). This rash characteristically does not fade under the pressure of a glass, the so-called glass test. A rash that doesn't fade in the test warrants swift medical attention.

When bacteria infect a cut in the skin, white blood cells travel into the skin from the bloodstream to fight the infection.

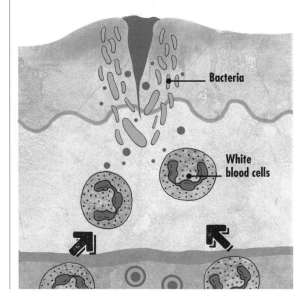

Bacteria

White blood cells

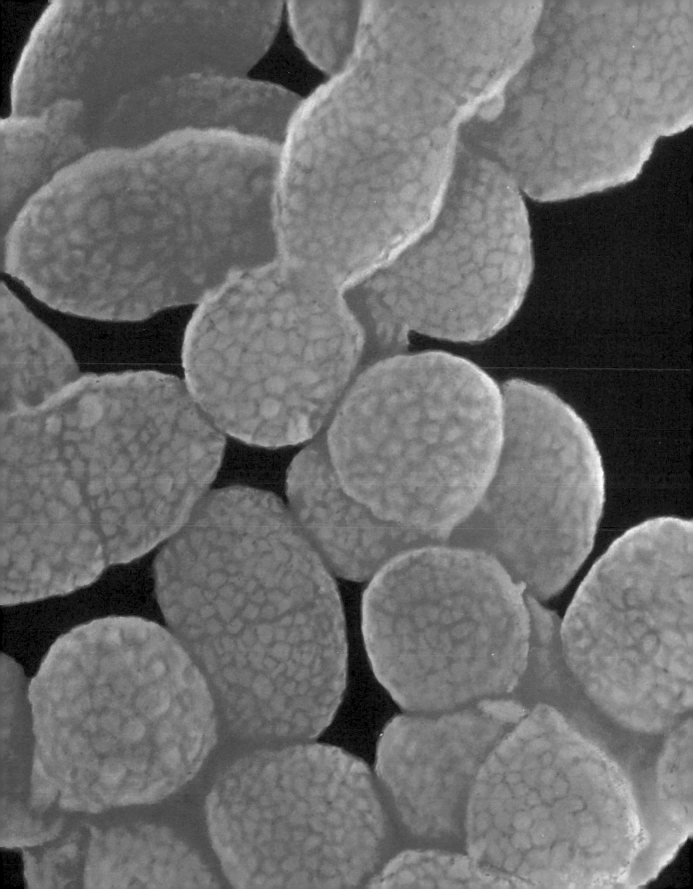

ACNE

Teenage acne starts out as pimples. These are formed, when the pores of the skin, which produce sweat, and those surrounding the hair follicles become clogged with sebum (skin oil) and dead skin. In these concealed niches, the anaerobic bacterium *Propionibacterium acnes* can dig its teeth in, leading to the inflamed spots of the more severe acne cases, particularly if the skin becomes too acidic.

However, it may not be that simple, as *P. acnes* is not the only bacteria associated with acnes, and it also lives on healthy skin. Doctors do not know exactly what causes acne, but some external factor is believed to tip the balance toward an outbreak. For example, acne patients have more, and more active, immune cells. The condition is more frequently seen in the industrial world, often lasting into adulthood.

It may, at least in part, be diet-related. Kitava, an island off the coast of Papua New Guinea is acne-free, a fact attributable to their Paleolithic diet. This consists of vegetables such as yams and sweet potatoes (which have a low GI or glycaemic index), high consumption of omega-3 fatty acids in tuna and fish eggs, and very few dairy products. Food for thought, and perhaps dietary action, on the acne front.

Antibiotics do work against acne, but possibly because of their systemic effect on the whole immune system. It may be all part of a picture of chronic inflammation, combined with an immune system that is hypersensitive to *P. acnes* or other skin bacteria. It is not just about the performance of one antibiotic or bacterium, but more about who is stealing from whom, how they are related to one another and whether they are happy about various relationship scenarios. Imbalances in our skin bacteria are not good for our skin health.

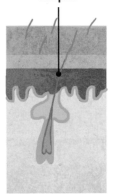

Healthy hair follicle and pore

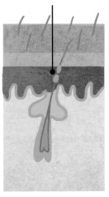

Sebum and dead skin

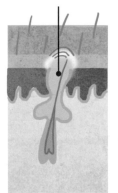

Bacterial infection and inflamation

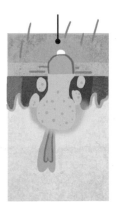

Acne

BACTERIAL TACTICS

Many skin bacteria have evolved tactics to deflect our immune response. For example, one of the traits of *Staphylococcus aureus* is its interference with the clotting process when it has invaded the skin, effectively placing the bacterium inside a blood clot and concealing it from the immune system. *Streptococcus pyogenes* produces two enzymes that destroy a key structural bond in antibodies, rendering them useless and so weakening the immune system. Targeting these enzymes is under investigation as a way of treating *S. pyogenes* infections.

BACTERIA ON THE MOVE

Many of our bacteria are harmless when sitting on the skin, but cause a problem if they get inside us. For example, *Staphylococcus epidermidis* is a very common skin commensal, but is also the most frequent cause of hospital-acquired infections on medical devices such as catheters or heart valves. They form biofilms on these that protect the bacteria from the immune system or antibiotics. *S. epidermidis* is increasingly resistant to antibiotics; it seems to be a reservoir of antibiotic-resistant genes that it can transfer to the closely related — but more virulent — organism, *S. aureus*.

Eating a Mediterranean diet promotes healthy skin by providing antioxidants to mop up damaging free radicals and via your fiber-hungry gut bacteria.

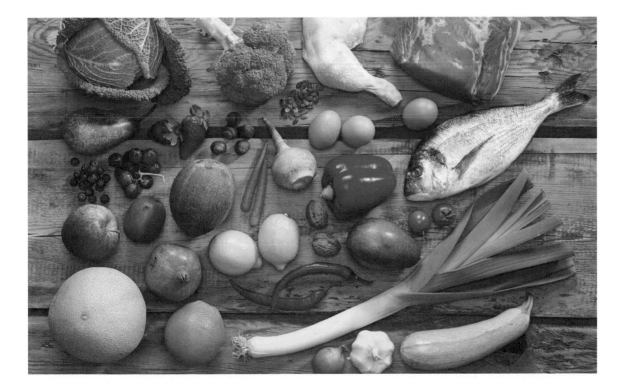

STAPHYLOCOCCUS

FIRST DOCUMENTED 1884

AUREUS

Staphylococcus aureus escaping destruction by human white blood cells (opposite page).

GRAM-POSITIVE COCCI

WHAT:
One of many *Staphylococcus* strains that populate the skin.

WHERE:
A normal inhabitant of skin, nose, mouth and throat, but one that can be a devil when excited.

HOW:
If the skin is broken, *Staphylococcus aureus* can start growing in the epidermal layer of the skin close to the point of entry, causing infections such as impetigo, boils and conjunctivitis or styes in the eye. *S. aureus* is also a cause of food poisoning. Growing on food, it releases an enterotoxin, a toxin that when eaten causes violent vomiting and diarrhea, thus ensuring the bacteria's spread to another unsuspecting host.

HISTORY:
S. aureus had a starring role in the discovery of the first antibiotic. In 1928 Alexander Fleming discovered that penicillin, produced by a fungus, inhibited the growth of *S. aureus*.

CASE NOTES:
S. aureus is one of the most virulent bacteria and its methicillin resistant form (MRSA) is now the scourge of many hospital wards. This superbug is very easily spread through human contact and causes a range of illnesses, from skin ailments to deadly diseases like pneumonia and meningitis. It is one of the ever-increasing number of bacteria that are resistant to antibiotics, and worldwide are responsible for ten million deaths a year.

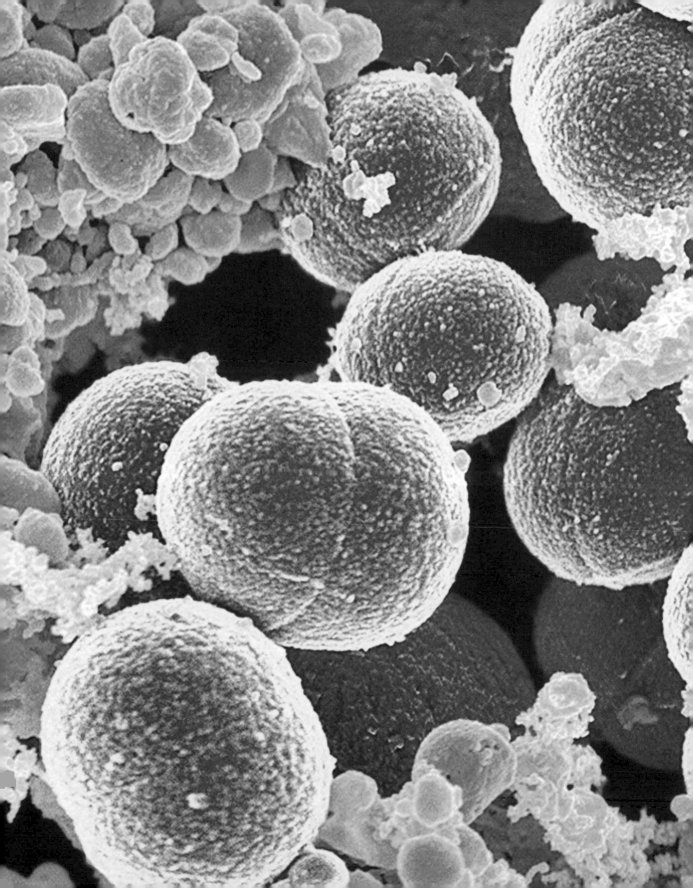

WHAT THE GOOD SKIN BACTERIA DO FOR US

Many of the bacteria on our skin are harmless — indeed, they work continuously to keep us healthy. Our commensal bacteria help to replenish the skin, replacing damaged and dying cells with new ones.

As in the gut, the sheer number of our helpful bacteria discourages the growth of other, more harmful bacteria by crowding out the bad guys. The good guys also stimulate the skin's immune responses to repel invasions of their more harmful colleagues — even sometimes killing these pathogenic bacteria.

Their assistance is more than skin deep. Bacteria perform vital tasks that the human genome has not evolved to do. Mice raised in germ-free conditions and that have no commensal skin bacteria are unable to fight off a parasitic infection. However, this immunity is miraculously restored when their skins are coated with the commensal bacterium *Staphylococcus epidermidis*.

BODY ODOR AND SEXUAL ATTRACTION

Sweat in our armpits is odorless: it only smells when our skin bacteria feast on the ammonia in the sweat. The precise scent produced depends on which bacteria you have on board. For example, *Corynebacterium* converts sweat into something that smells like onions and testosterone into something that smells like vanilla, urine or nothing, depending on the subject's genes.

Sexual attraction through pheromones also comes into the equation here. Female students at the University of Bern, in Switzerland, were given T-shirts worn by male students and asked to rate them in order of attractiveness. The women selected the shirts of men whose immune system varied most from their own, thereby increasing the possibility of producing healthy children.

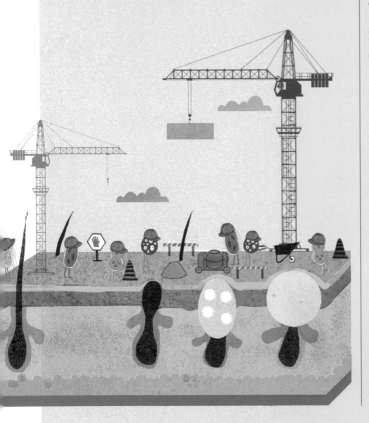

Beneficial bacteria labor to deter pathogens by competing for nutrients and stimulating the immune system.

PROPIONIBACTERIUM

FIRST DOCUMENTED 1902

ACNES

GRAM-POSITIVE ROD

WHAT:
Despite its implied role in the development of types of acne, this is a commensal bacterium, part of our normal healthy skin flora.

WHERE:
This bacteria colonizes the sebaceous glands all over the skin, but particularly on the face and upper back, and makes enzymes that degrade the fats within sebum.

HOW:
The free fatty acids that are released both help *S. acnes'* adherence to the skin and contribute to the acidic pH of the skin surface.

CASE NOTES:
Many of the common pathogenic bacteria such as *Staphylococcus aureus* and *Streptococcus pyogenes* are inhibited by an acidic pH. A pH of around 5.0 is just right for our helpful bacteria and there are steps you can take to maintain that (see page 68).

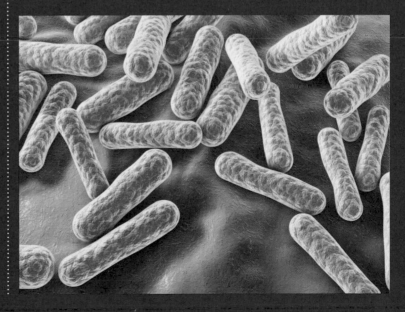

Propionibacterium acnes bacteria

STAPHYLOCOCCUS

FIRST DOCUMENTED 1884

EPIDERMIDIS

GRAM-POSITIVE COCCI

CASE NOTES:
Beware — this is an opportunistic pathogen. In people with a weakened immune system, it can cause infections, for example in catheters or artificial heart valves.

HISTORY:
Research on this bacteria is part of a growing body of evidence that links commensal skin bacteria with guiding our immune responses to target the bad guys.

Staphylococcus epidermidis
(red) embedded in a complex carbohydrate matrix, similar to that found in the skin (yellow).

WHAT:
S. epidermidis is the most commonly isolated bacteria on human skin. It is definitely one to encourage, but only if it's in the right place (see page 61).

WHERE:
Found all over the skin so not a species that you can specifically promote, just one to celebrate when it is in a good mood.

HOW:
It has a secret weapon, an enzyme that inhibits the growth of skin pathogens such as *Staphylococcus aureus* and some of the *Streptococcus* species, both of which cause infections. And cross talk between *Staphylococcus epidermidis* and skin cells helps skin cell survival and repair during infections.

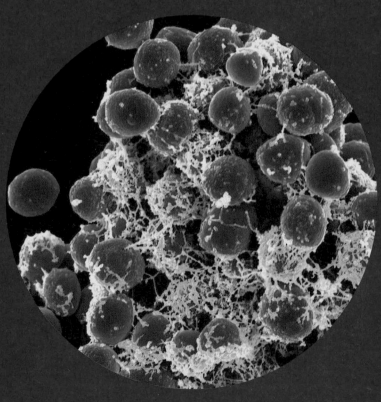

MAKING BACTERIA WORK FOR OUR SKIN

Scientists are increasingly finding ways to harness the properties of bacteria to help skin health. These range from bacteria used by the cosmetic industry (Botox) to dermatologists' focus on skin cancer.

Many of the symptoms of bacterial infections actually result from bacterial toxins. One such toxin, Botox — the botulinum toxin of *Clostridium botulinum* — paralyses muscles, removing wrinkles that are caused by muscle contractions. Less well publicized are its medical uses: to treat eye disorders or to control sweating and migraines. With its frequent application, in miniscule quantities, for cosmetic and medical procedures, it is easy to forget what a toxic substance Botox is. One gram is thought to be sufficient to kill one million people.

Protecting the skin from the damaging effects of the sun's ultraviolet (UV) rays plays an important role in avoiding skin cancer. UV radiation triggers the mutations in DNA which lead to malignant melanomas. In 2013, Norwegian researchers discovered a bacteria in the Norwegian Sea with a unique characteristic. *Micrococcus luteus* contains a pigment that has the ability to absorb UV radiation. Scientists are now trying to increase the production of this super sunscreen for use in sun creams.

IN PRAISE OF ALCOHOL

Alcohol in the form of hand sprays or gels is a valuable weapon in the fight against disease. In workplaces and hospitals they are even effective against hardy and virulent pathogens such as MRSA. Anti-bacterial agents are less effective than alcohol, which kills a higher proportion of bacteria. The alcohol breaks down the bacterial cell membrane and then destroys bacterial proteins inside the cell. Recent studies have suggested that these alcohol-containing sprays or gels work best on clean hands. Removing the dirt that bacteria cling to allows the alcohol easy access to kill the remaining bacteria. Rubbing the gel rigorously into the skin for as long as possible, at least 30 seconds, is also important. Sprays containing at least 70 percent alcohol will kill a similar percentage of bacteria but the effects are short-lived, so regular application of alcohol gels is recommended.

Botox, the botulinum toxin, is derived from the Clostridium botulinum bacterium and can be injected into people for cosmetic and medical purposes.

ENCOURAGING THE GOOD AND DISCOURAGING THE BAD

Providing a convenient living space for a diverse population of health-promoting bacteria is the name of the game. If you allow bad bacteria too much room and the right environmental conditions, there is less incentive for good bacteria to hang around.

Scientists are only beginning fully to characterize the bacteria that live on our skin and the conditions that affect the balance of good and bad bacteria. We can now start to look for answers to a whole series of questions. How do ethnicity, lifestyles, geographical location, gender, age, weather conditions, diet, skin pH, antibiotics or creams applied to the skin — cosmetic or medical — affect the skin microbiome?

The pH of the skin is one area where there's some certainty, with the term "pH-balanced" more than just a marketing slogan. Every time we wash or use soaps, the skin's pH is raised from its natural state of around 5.0. Washing is obviously important to remove harmful pathogens, but current advice is not to overuse harsh soaps and cleansers. Even plain tap water, with a pH of around 8.0, raises skin pH and makes it harder for our beneficial bacteria to hang on.

Getting some exercise in the fresh air, such as walks or gardening, exposes us to a wide range of beneficial bacteria. Clothing may make a difference too; natural fibers such as cotton and linen support a more normal balance of skin bacteria than synthetic fibers. Drying clothes outside also encourages a balanced bacterial population,

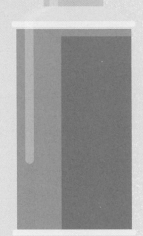

AOB spray is now being tested to see how reintroducing these beneficial bacteria affects our skin health.

ready to be transferred onto your skin the next time you wear those clothes.

UV light from the sun varies significantly across longitude and latitude, but may also influence our skin bacteria. The application of UV light is being developed as an anti-bacterial treatment, for example in the disinfection of wounds in surgery, and it is probable that studies of geographical location will reveal differing levels of commensal bacteria.

A SKIN-FRIENDLY DIET

A Mediterranean-style diet (see page 113) will benefit your overall health and your skin health. Some of these are direct effects; for example, olives and their oil, contain Vitamin E, which increases skin suppleness. Brightly colored vegetables contain antioxidants that mop up damaging free radicals that can harm skin cells and other cells in the body. Other effects are mediated by feeding fiber to the gut bacteria, allowing the release of fatty acids and vitamins which are essential for skin health.

WASHING WELL

The skin on the hands, unlike elsewhere on the body, is in regular contact with potential pathogens. Care should be taken to avoid transferring bacteria from places where they belong (in the feces, for example) to places where they do not, such as the mouth or eyes. Keeping pathogens at bay is not a new problem. Ever since the 1860s, when Joseph Lister introduced sterile techniques in his hospital, cleaning protocols have helped to control the spread of pathogens. Simple measures such as hand-washing save lives.

Most people do not wash their hands long enough; if you are unsure sing "Happy Birthday" to yourself,

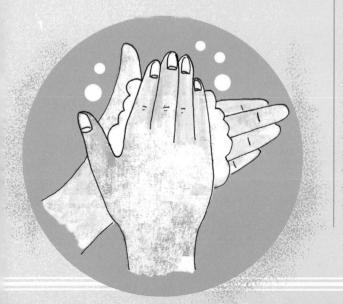

LESS IS MORE

Be careful not to overuse cosmetics. A recent survey of the metabolites on human faces found that a regular barrage of beauty products drowns out natural microbial molecules, which help to regulate skin growth and our immune response.

twice. That only takes about 25 seconds, but is sufficient to remove the stickiest of pathogenic bacteria and prevent at least one-third of cases of diarrhea.

When you wash your hands properly, with warm water and soap, you are not killing bacteria. The soap and temperature of the water just help to physically remove the dirt, dead skin or skin oils to which the bacteria are clinging.

BRINGING BACTERIA BACK

Our modern obsession with cleanliness in daily life has seen a backlash in some quarters. David Whitlock (no relation) founded a biotech company called AOBiome in 2013 in Cambridge, Massachusetts. A chemical engineer who had studied soil microbes, he is part of a movement to increase our skin health by putting beneficial bacteria back, rather than stripping them away. Whitlock has not showered for 12 years, relying instead on a twice weekly sponge down: his family and friends are still happy to get close and his beneficial skin bacteria are finding their feet again. Ammonia oxidizing bacteria (AOB) are from this beneficial group. These are common in nature but, despite their known beneficial effects on the skin, are slow to repopulate after washing. Whitlock's cosmetic spray may be the answer.

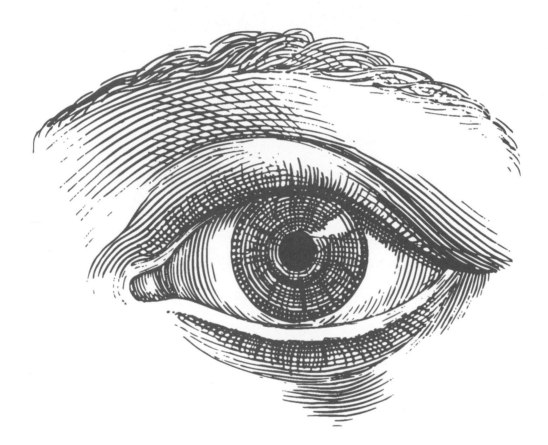

THE EYE

Bacterial eye infections are common, but for years it was thought that healthy eyes were a no-go area for bacteria. Modern research is now telling a different story.

WHERE AND HOW BACTERIA LIVE IN OUR EYES

The 2008 human microbiome project did not feature the eye, as it was one of the body sites that was presumed to be sterile and bacteria-free. In 2014, however, scientists began to present the findings from the Ocular Microbiome project — mapping the DNA of bacteria found on the eye. To their surprise, they found that bacteria do live on heathy eyes, mainly on the conjunctiva, but there is a much lower diversity than in other areas of the body and lower overall numbers: tens of species rather than hundreds or thousands.

The inner compartment of the eye certainly sees little bacterial action. Here, there is a special relationship with the immune system, known as immune privilege. Thanks to a combination of physical barriers (the blood–retina barrier), and clever action on the part of the immune system, the inner compartment of the eye is able to keep the outside world at bay.

In contrast, the external compartment is constantly exposed to bacteria in our environment, so it is quite surprising that the eye does not get more bacterial infections. The relentless mechanical action of blinking and our protective tear film, not to mention humans' unique ability to shed tears, all help to keep those pathogenic bacteria at a distance. Tears contain an enzyme called lysozyme which is a pretty efficient bacterial killer. The hostile environment of the eye's surface probably explains why bacterial numbers and diversity are low.

Bacteria that live on the healthy eye are often equally at home in other sites in the body. Like elsewhere, much of the colonization takes place at or just after birth (see pages 132–33). The most commonly detected bacteria are *Corynebacterium* (see page 77), also abundant in the nose and skin. Some strains of the commensal eye bacteria, such as *Streptococcus*, are also found in the mouth.

Perhaps not surprisingly, given their fondness for exploring noses and mouths, young children have a higher bacterial diversity in their eyes. By the same token, eye infections are more prevalent in children. In general, eye bacterial infections start when there has been some damage or irritation to the eye's surface. One of the most common of the bacterial pathogens, *Pseudomonas aeruginosa* (see page 75), is picked up from our surroundings. A bacterial infection elsewhere in the body may sometimes trigger disease, for example in the case of uveitis (inflammation of the eye's middle layer). Most bacteria are found on the conjunctiva, the membrane that covers the front of the eye and lines the inside of the eyelids.

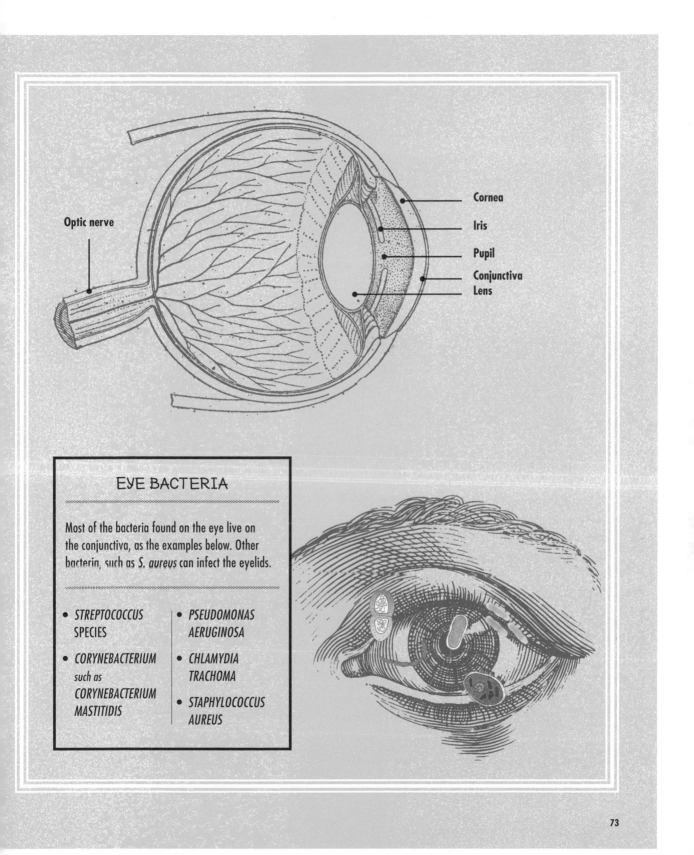

Optic nerve

Cornea

Iris

Pupil

Conjunctiva

Lens

EYE BACTERIA

Most of the bacteria found on the eye live on the conjunctiva, as the examples below. Other bacteria, such as *S. aureus* can infect the eyelids.

- *STREPTOCOCCUS SPECIES*
- *CORYNEBACTERIUM* such as *CORYNEBACTERIUM MASTITIDIS*
- *PSEUDOMONAS AERUGINOSA*
- *CHLAMYDIA TRACHOMA*
- *STAPHYLOCOCCUS AUREUS*

EYE BACTERIAL INFECTIONS

Bacterial eye diseases are prevalent worldwide and include conjunctivitis, styes and trachoma. Other bacterial infections, such as those that cause inflammation in the joints, can enter the body via the eye.

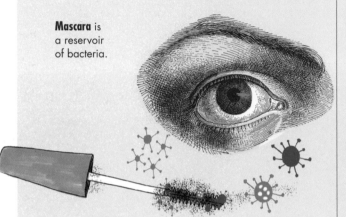

Mascara is a reservoir of bacteria.

In conjunctivitis, or "pink eye," the clear membrane covering the front of the eyeball becomes infected. The conjunctiva flows back behind the eye and forms the inside surface of the eyelids. Its continuity keeps objects such as eyelashes and contact lenses from irretrievably sliding behind your eyeball: they cannot get "lost." But at the same time, the conjunctiva is loose enough to allow free eye movement.

Some conjunctivitis is caused by a virus or the symptoms of hay fever. However, bacteria such as *Staphylococcus aureus* (see page 62) and *Pseudomonas aeruginosa* are two principal culprits.

If pus is present, indicating a bacterial infection, antibiotic eye drops can help. Otherwise it is important just to keep eyes clean (see pages 78–79) while this self-limiting infection clears up.

Strictly speaking, styes are not a disease of the eye itself, but are associated with poor eye hygiene. They occur when an eyelash follicle or sweat gland on the inside or the outside of the eyelid become infected. A painful red lump then forms. As with conjunctivitis, *Staphylococcus aureus* is very often the culprit.

Antibiotics are not recommended for styes, as there is little evidence that they are effective. Usually styes get better on their own. A warm compress may be all that is needed: a clean face cloth soaked in recently boiled, but lukewarm water soothes and helps to release the pus. Simple saline solutions are good too. The old tradition of rubbing a wedding ring on the eyelid should also be avoided, as it may introduce other pathogenic bacteria into an already inflamed environment, causing more problems. Compounds that contain gold do have well-known antibacterial properties, from which this tradition may have originated, but the gold in a wedding ring is inert and unlikely to help.

Trachoma is a very nasty eye disease which, although not common in the U.S. or the U.K., affects 41 countries around the world and results in visual impairment or blindness in 1.9 million people. It is caused by the bacteria *Chlamydia trachomatis* (see page 112), which has the dubious accolade of being top of the leader-board for damaging infectious eye diseases. It is also a major player in sexually transmitted diseases.

PSEUDOMONAS
FIRST
DOCUMENTED
1882
AERUGINOSA

GRAM-NEGATIVE ROD

WHAT:

P. aeruginosa is a free-living bacterium usually found in soil and water.

HOW:

P. aeruginosa is a highly skilled opportunistic pathogen which exploits a break in our defenses to initiate an infection. It almost never infects undamaged areas, yet there is hardly any site in the body that it cannot infect, given the chance. In the eye, *P. aeruginosa* causes conjunctivitis; elsewhere it is responsible for respiratory, gastrointestinal and urinary tract infections.

WHERE:

It can grow anywhere, favoring moist places and having very basic nutritional requirements. The wet surface of the eye is perfect.

CASE NOTES:

P. aeruginosa is a tough cookie, resistant to many antiseptics and antibiotics. It is one of the most successful bad bacteria we know.

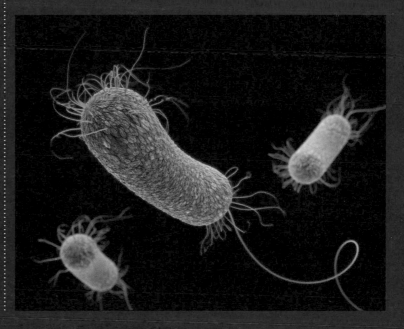

Pseudomonas aeruginosa bacterium showing the flagella used for motility.

WHAT THE GOOD EYE BACTERIA DO FOR US

Now we know that bacteria live on the surface of a healthy eye, we need to ask what they are doing there. It is likely that, as in other sites of the body, these good bacteria outnumber the bad, helping to keep the latter under control and influencing the immune system, but it is still largely unclear how it all works.

Does the surface of the eye have long-term residents, as other moist surfaces such as the gut do? Or does the continuous blinking and tears mean there is a regular turnover? Are the small numbers of good bacteria really enough to influence the bad guys — particularly when a pathogenic bacterium finds its way in?

We do have some leads on the good bacteria's role If you are unlucky enough to contract a bacterial infection it helps if your eyes are awash with good bacteria. People with reduced levels of commensal bacteria tend to have more severe eye infections than those with a greater diversity of bacteria and high numbers of good bacteria compared with the pathogenic kind.

Corynebacterium and *Streptococcus* can promote the immune responses to pathogens such as *P. aeruginosa* by recruiting neutrophils — a type of white blood cell in the immune system. Neutrophils loiter with intent, poised to kill bacterial intruders.

In 2017 scientists studying the eyes of animals showed for the first time that a bacterium, *Corynebacterium mastitidis*, was acquired from the mother at birth. Not only was *C. mastitidis* a long-term resident of the eye, but it also earned its keep by stimulating several arms of the immune response to repel pathogens. Now scientists are expecting to find other long-term residents, not just bacteria that have "crash-landed" from invading fingers. If *C. mastitidis* or any other commensal bacteria are found to perform the same function in human eyes, they could be used to inoculate against diseases such as conjunctivitis.

Antibiotic eye drops can treat bacterial eye infections.

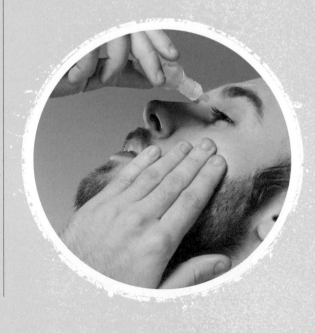

CORYNEBACTERIUM
FIRST DOCUMENTED 1997
MASTITIDIS

GRAM-POSITIVE ROD

WHAT:
C. mastitidis is part of an extremely diverse group of bacteria including animal and plant pathogens.

WHERE:
C. mastitidis is found on the surface of the eye.

HOW:
C. mastitidis has gained newfound fame as a friend to the immune system. For example, it induces the production of a key molecule secreted by T cells that is involved in protecting against infections.

C. diphtheriae, a close relative of *C. mastitidis*, shares the rod shape of the latter.

CASE NOTES:
Nearly one hundred Corynebacteria species are clinically relevant to humans.

C. mastitidis has until recently been eclipsed by its better known family member *C. diphtheriae*, the highly pathogenic bacteria that causes the disease diphtheria.

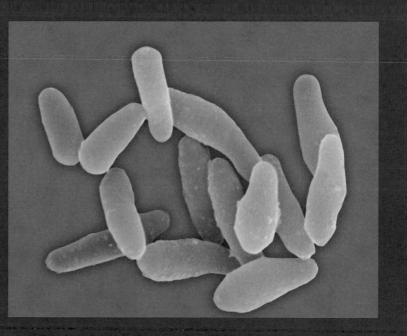

ENCOURAGING THE GOOD AND DISCOURAGING THE BAD

Less is more where the eye is concerned. The less interference, and therefore the fewer opportunities to introduce pathogenic bacteria, the more diverse (and helpful) bacteria will be in evidence.

The skin also has a big role: clean hands mean clean eyes. Where possible, steering clear of anyone else with a bacterial infection is a good tactic too.

However, hand hygiene is not the whole picture. Keeping a diverse population of bacteria on the eye is likely to be important — particularly as many pathogenic bacteria are increasingly resistant to the natural antibacterial action of the tears or antibiotic treatments. These bad bacteria thus have a distinct edge over other bacteria on the hostile surface of the eye.

Contact lens wearers should take particular care. Bacterial infections of the cornea affect 7 to 25 percent of wearers, possibly because they have a low diversity of good bacteria and are therefore more prone to infections. The surface of contact lenses seems to provide a particularly favorable location for pathogenic species such as *Staphylococcus*.

Scientists in Australia have recently developed antibacterial contact lenses. This prototype is in its infancy, but they appear as safe and effective as regular lenses and they discourage the growth of the major pathogens *Pseudomonas* and *Staphylococcus aureus*. Keep an eye out for it!

Contact lens wearers have more contact with their eyes than non-lens wearers, so it is important that hands are clean. Daily disposable lenses are the most hygienic, avoiding any problems that may occur in cleaning or storing other kinds of lenses.

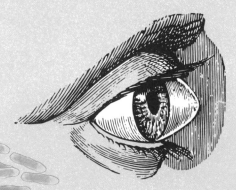
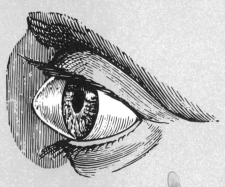

Keep your eyes healthy with good hand hygiene, particularly if you wear contact lenses.

BRIGHT EYES

If you have an eye infection or are prone to them, the following tips will help to discourage bad bacteria from finding a home:

DO wash your hands well with warm soapy water. Remove eye make-up before bed and replace eye make-up every six months. Keep eyelids and eyelashes clean. Wash pillowcases, towels and face cloths regularly in hot water and detergent.

If your eye is infected, wipe any pus from the corners of the eye with a clean cotton swab, moistened in cool, recently boiled water.

DO NOT share towels, rub the eyes or insert contact lenses if you have not recently washed your hands.

healthy eyes, the most prominent strain being the pathogen *Pseudomonas*. Researchers found that this decrease in diversity occurred before the eye infection was evident. Monitoring what bacteria are living on your eye could help to prevent bacterial infections by providing a window of opportunity to enable you to intervene.

Antibiotics are a vital line of defense against bacterial infections, but the penalty of getting rid of the bad bacteria is the damage done to the good. Future approaches to bacterial infections are likely to include probiotic eye drops, introducing helpful bacteria into the eye. An early study with eye drops containing *Lactobacillus* has shown promising results in conjunctivitis patients.

AN EYE-FRIENDLY DIET

Eating a Mediterranean-style diet (see page 113) benefits eyes. Many of the vitamins and minerals found in these foods are essential for eye health. For example, the mineral zinc, which is found in turkey, sardines and nuts such as cashews, has a proven role in helping the immune system deal with the bacteria that cause complaints such as conjunctivitis and styes.

SEEING A WAY FORWARD

Research is now focused on finding out what the bacteria on the eye do and how important it is to promote a diverse range of commensal bacteria. In cases of keratitis, an infection of the cornea, the bacterial diversity drops to about half that in

SHAKE UP YOUR MAKE-UP

Old make-up is a haven for bacteria. Mascara is the worst offender, but keep an eye on liquid eyeliner too. Both provide a perfect level of moisture for bacterial growth, and regular applications ensure that unfriendly bacteria get every opportunity to infect the eye. It is recommended that you change make-up every year, and mascara every six months. Regular washing of make-up brushes and nightly removal of make-up will also help to keep bad bacteria at bay. A 27-year-old Australian women lived to regret sharing a friend's make-up brush when she picked up a methicillin-resistant *Staphylococcus aureus* infection from it. The bacterium attacked her spine and left her paralysed and in a wheel chair. Thankfully, such scare stories are rare.

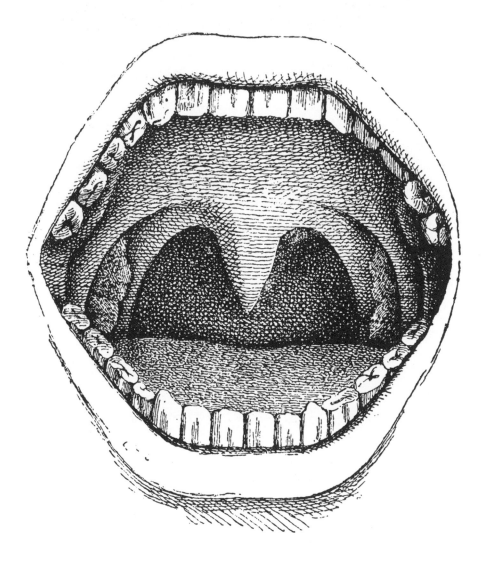

THE MOUTH

What goes on in our mouths matters: our oral health depends on our mouth bacteria, and it does not end there. We open the door to bacteria whenever we breathe, eat or drink. From birth, the average person swallows around a million bacteria in every mouthful of food.

WHERE AND HOW BACTERIA LIVE IN OUR MOUTH

The mouth provides a cozy home to at least six billion bacteria. It contains a number of different habitats, including the teeth, the gums, tongue, hard and soft palates and the tonsils. The environment is warm and nutrient-rich; it is also continuously bathed with saliva, which has a mainly neutral pH.

Subtle differences, such as pH values and varying food availability, affect which bacteria live in these different habitats. Over 700 different species of bacteria can live here, although most people host only about 50 different varieties, with *Streptococcus* species predominating. Many mouth bacteria are harmless or even beneficial, helping to digest food and keep our gums and teeth healthy.

Although each person has a unique bacterial profile, researchers have recently discovered that it is possible to group mouth bacteria along ethnic lines. The similar species profile in each group — Caucasian, Chinese, Latino or African-American — was attributed to their shared genes. Bacteria under the gum line had the strongest correlation to ethnicity, probably because bacteria here are the least disrupted by environmental influences, such as smoking and diet.

Nobody really understands how our genes influence our mouth bacteria, but studies in twins confirm that our predisposition to certain bacteria may be inherited; it remains even when twins live apart.

On one side are dental plaque, a sticky, colorless film of bacteria, plus sugary food and drinks. The bacteria use these to produce acid, which eats away at the tooth. On the other side are the minerals in our saliva and food (calcium and phosphate), plus fluoride in toothpaste and water that help tooth enamel repair itself.

Among the main bacteria living in both healthy and diseased mouths are species traditionally viewed as "bad," such as *Streptococcus mutans*, *Porphyromonas gingivalis* and *Streptococcus pyogenes*, while the "good" include *S. oralis*, *S. sanguinis* and *S. salivarius*. Other bacteria can happily play for both sides, depending on the pitch conditions. For example, *Fusobacterium nucleatum* (FAD-1) has some attractive features, but is also associated with gum disease and a raft of serious diseases elsewhere in the body.

MOUTH BACTERIA

The mouth provides a wealth of different habitats and conditions for bacteria, including:

1. GUMS:
   PORPHYROMONAS GINGIVALIS

2. SOFT PALATE:
   STREPTOCOCCUS SPECIES like *S. ORALIS, S. SANGUINIS* and *S. SALIVARIUS*

3. TONGUE:
   FUSOBACTERIUM NUCLEATUM

4. TEETH:
   STREPTOCOCCUS MUTANS

5. TONSILS:
   STREPTOCOCCUS PYOGENES.

Gums

Hard palate

Soft palate

Uvula

Tonsil

Tongue

Teeth

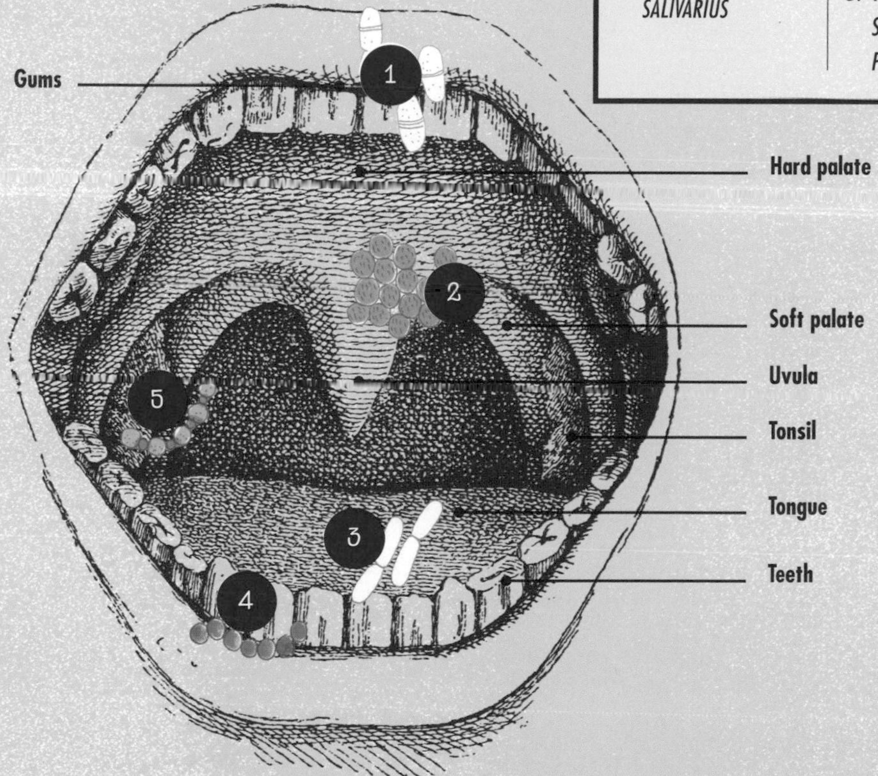

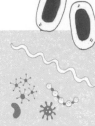

MOUTH BACTERIAL INFECTIONS

Scientists now think the word pathogenic is overused in terms of the mouth. It suggests that bacteria should not be there at all, but the reality is that so-called "bad" bacteria may always be there, just keeping a low profile. We know that our commensal mouth bacteria are essential for maintaining a healthy mouth, but that the balance may sometimes be shifted in favor of bacteria causing tooth decay, gum disease or sore throats.

Changes in pH and diet are the two main drivers of the descent into disease. A diet high in sugar causes a drop in pH, and the acidic mouth this produces offers a haven to bacteria such as *Streptococcus mutans*, while neutral pH-loving bacteria are displaced. Soft foods high in carbohydrate, such as bread and chips, get trapped between the teeth; regular brushing and flossing is required to remove this handy reservoir of food for hungry bacteria.

TOOTH DECAY

Tooth extraction because of decay has become a problem over recent years in many countries, sometimes resulting in hospital admissions even for children under ten. The bacteria *S. mutans* and sugary drinks are behind this alarming trend. *S. mutans* is the king of decay; it is present throughout the mouth, but causes problems principally on the teeth, feeding on sugar; the by-product of its ravenous appetite is enamel-eroding acid, the main cause of tooth decay. However, regular brushing, and ditching sugary drinks and snacks, will discourage its growth and destructive action.

GUM DISEASE (GINGIVITIS)

Porphyromonas gingivalis is commonly associated with gum disease, something that affects at least 50 percent of adults. The toxins of *P. gingivalis* disrupt the harmony of the protective bacteria in the mouth. Bacteria such as *P. gingivalis* are able to sneak in beneaththe gum line, and the resulting inflammation and swelling can lead to telltale signs of bleeding as you brush your teeth. When the infection takes hold, the bone and connective tissue in and around the teeth are affected, eventually leading to periodontal disease and tooth loss. There is also a proven connection between gum disease and cardiovascular disease, possibly because the inflammatory molecules and activated immune cells travel in the bloodstream to damage the heart.

STREP THROAT

The most common bacterial infection of the throat is strep throat, caused by *Streptococcus pyogenes* (see page 86); it results in a red, inflamed throat and tonsils, with characteristic white patches of pus. Many people carry this bacteria in their throats but when the immune system is compromised it can take a stronger hold. Handwashing minimizes spread and antibiotics can treat the infection.

PORPHYROMONAS GINGIVALIS

FIRST DOCUMENTED 1980

GRAM-NEGATIVE ROD

P. gingivalis may be a "keystone pathogen" that co-opts other bacteria into the destructive process. Scientists have shown that *P. gingivalis* initiates an inflammatory immune response that destroys bone. The breakdown of the bone provides food for other bacteria to continue their destructive work. Various plant extracts, such as polyphenols from rhubarb roots, are being investigated for their antibacterial effects against *P. gingivalis.*

Porphyromonas gingivailis

WHAT:
P. gingivalis is a secondary colonizer, meaning that it needs another bacterium to hang on to. It uses one of the *Streptococcus* species as a primary colonizer.

WHERE:
The bacterium is found in over 80 percent of gum plaque samples from patients with chronic gum disease.

HOW:
P. gingivalis relies on the fermentation of amino acids, a property that helps it survive deep in the gum and tooth pockets where sugar availability is low. The enzymes the bacterium uses, called proteases, break down the gums and teeth; they also make the bacteria very resistant to the body's immune defense mechanisms.

STREPTOCOCCUS

FIRST DOCUMENTED 1909

SALIVARIUS

GRAM-POSITIVE COCCI

WHAT:
A commensal bacteria that colonizes the mouth and upper respiratory tract, usually in a chain formation, hours after birth.

WHERE:
The K12 strain of *S. salivarius* was isolated in 2004 from the saliva of a healthy schoolchild who had a large quantity of this bacteria, together with a long history of no throat infections.

HOW:
S. salivarius K12 can combat sore throats or tonsillitis caused by *S. pyrogenes*. The bacterium might also make bad breath a thing of the past.

CASE NOTES:
S. salivarius K12 has been used in New Zealand as an oral probiotic for over ten years. As the first successful probiotic for mouth and throat health, *S. salivarius* is available in the U.S. and online in the form of tablets and chewing gums.

STREPTOCOCCUS

FIRST DOCUMENTED 1874

PYOGENES

GRAM-POSITIVE COCCI

WHAT:
An anaerobic bacterium, which is an opportunistic pathogen.

WHERE:
Sticks to receptors on the surface of cells using an adherence protein called M protein.

HOW:
Produces multiple toxins such as streptolysins, which destroy red blood cells, and leukocidins, which kill white blood cells. The resulting pus explains the bacteria's name: pyogenic means "pus-forming."

CASE NOTES:
Causes multiples diseases ranging from the mild, such as impetigo and strep throat, to the more severe, such as scarlet fever, rheumatic fever and toxic shock syndrome. Since the advent of antibiotics, fatalities from these diseases are now fortunately rare.

WHAT THE GOOD MOUTH BACTERIA DO FOR US

Many of the bacteria in our mouths are harmless or even beneficial, helping to digest food and keep our gums and teeth healthy.

The digestion of food starts in the mouth and bacteria get their teeth in here too. Sometimes the results are negative, as the digestion of sugars leads to tooth decay, but sometimes the results are good. For instance, the production of nitric oxide, which helps to control blood pressure, starts with the action of mouth bacteria on the nitrates in vegetables.

Helpful bacteria also keep the immune system focused on any threatening behavior from bad bacteria, sending out signals not to overreact.

When bacteria touch base with the epithelial cells lining our mouths, they can produce antimicrobial peptides. These molecules, nature's natural antibiotics, kill bacteria, as well as destroying fungi and some viruses. One of these peptides, produced by *Fusobacterium nucleatum* and called FAD-1, has been isolated by scientists and is being developed to target specific areas of the mouth where infection is difficult to control.

A newly discovered species of *Streptococcus*, designated A12, was isolated from healthy teeth in 2016 and shown to produce copious quantities of hydrogen peroxide — a substance that is deadly to the tooth-decay culprit *S. mutans*. The A12 strain also prevented *S. mutans* from using its antibacterial toxins to kill other bacteria, such as the good guy *Streptococcus sanguinis*. Packaging good bacteria such as *Streptococcus* A12 in a pill might be a future way to maintain a healthy mouth. Measuring the levels of such bacteria could also provide a risk assessment for tooth decay.

Even the long roots of adult teeth can lose their grip on our gums if bacterial infections cause significant tooth or bone decay and gum disease.

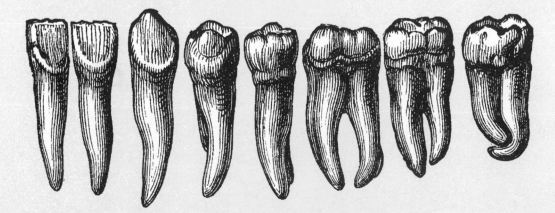

ENCOURAGING THE GOOD AND DISCOURAGING THE BAD

In terms of oral health, a mouth where predominantly good bacteria dominate as part of a balanced bacterial community is the ideal. Once you have acquired a strain of oral bacteria, you are unlikely to get rid of it. Bacteria living together in a complex, interacting community means that any individual bacterium may have different properties than one living in isolation. Such interdependence means that even if we eliminate just one species, this may affect others.

The good news is that you can manage and control the bacteria in your mouth. The twice-daily use of — and regular changes of — toothbrushes, plus flossing, are important ways of removing a food source for bacteria, such as sugar coating the teeth or food trapped between the teeth. Antibiotics are still used regularly to treat tooth infections, but modern oral health products, from lozenges to mouthwashes, are designed to optimize the balance of bacteria in the mouth.

Oral probiotics have become a hot topic. These often focus on bacteria that have evolved to operate optimally in the mouth. Mint lozenges containing *Bacillus coagulans* and *S. salivarius* can inhibit the formation of biofilms by *S. mutans*, responsible for much tooth decay, while leaving the rest of the microbiome intact. Toothpastes are also being developed that contain a protective *Lactobacillus* strain and chemicals that inhibit bacteria.

Mouthwashes are also popular for the introduction of antibacterial agents, such as chlorhexidine. Probiotic mouthwashes are still in development, but the results are encouraging: the bacterial strains used in trials, such as *S. salivarius*,

ON THE MENU

WATER: drinking water can help to clean your teeth; a quick gargle is as effective as mouthwash at removing pathogenic bacteria

TEA (green and black): contain polyphenols, chemicals that interact with plaque bacteria and stop them growing or producing acid

RAW ONION: researchers in Korea have shown that raw onions eradicate four strains of bacteria that cause tooth decay and gum disease

APPLES, CARROTS AND CELERY: these are dental detergents and any food that gets saliva flowing is good. Next to good home dental care, this is your best natural defense against tooth decay and gum disease. Apples also contain xylitol, which inhibits acid production

WASABI: Research in Japan has found this spicy condiment can stop bacteria from sticking to your teeth

outcompeted the bad bacteria that cause tooth decay, gum disease and throat infection. The whitening effect of the hydrogen peroxide could even lead to a pearly white smile. New therapies for gum disease include amixicile, an antibacterial agent that has two major advantages over conventional antibiotic therapy: it inhibits an enzyme pathway that is not commonly found in our beneficial bacteria, and its use may not lead to drug resistance.

A MOUTH-FRIENDLY DIET

Skulls from before the 16th century, when the main sweetener in diet was honey, show very little evidence of tooth decay. Honey has antimicrobial properties, in contrast to processed sugars that provide food for bacteria such as S. *mutans*, a major cause of tooth decay. Avoid these sugars and make sure that you have some healthy food on the menu

— beneficial to your overall as well as oral health. Many foodstuffs encourage the production of saliva, good for both our teeth and breath. Bad breath is caused by hydrogen sulfide, or bad egg gas, produced when bacteria in your mouth feast on leftovers from the day's food. The condition is particularly bad first thing in the morning, as saliva production is largely switched off at night and bacterial numbers rise. The most common cause of bad breath is poor oral hygiene, but it can also be caused by smoking, gut problems, diseases such as diabetes or certain medications.

SMOKING

It is no secret that smoking is bad for your lungs and your cardiovascular health, but it turns out to be not great for your mouth either. Smoking lowers the pH of your mouth and, as cigarette smoke decreases the availability of oxygen, it enables acid-loving, anaerobic bacteria such as S.*mutans* to flourish. Vaping is likely to be better, but electronic cigarettes still contain nicotine, which inhibits saliva production.

Bacterial numbers fluctuate during the day, depending on the availability of food in the mouth. After meal times, levels rise, peaking at night when saliva production is low.

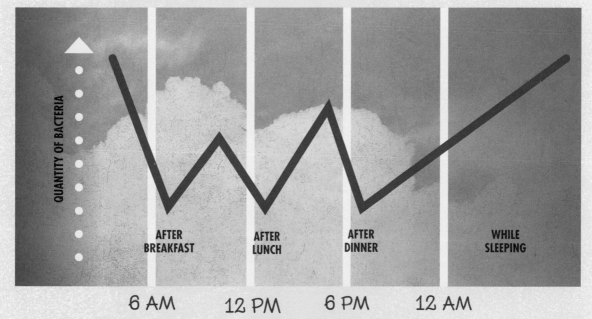

QUANTITY OF BACTERIA

AFTER BREAKFAST · AFTER LUNCH · AFTER DINNER · WHILE SLEEPING

6 AM · 12 PM · 6 PM · 12 AM

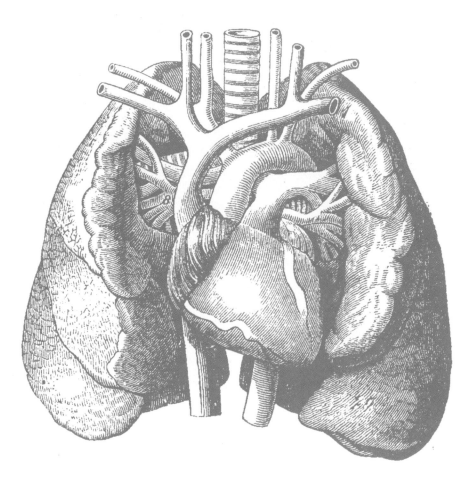

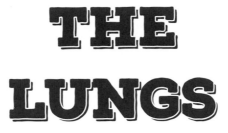

THE LUNGS

Every breath we take exposes the respiratory tract leading down to the lungs to bacteria. Although far less populated than the mouth community that feeds it, the lung microbiome has a key role to play in our respiratory health.

WHERE AND HOW BACTERIA LIVE IN OUR LUNGS

As gatekeeper to the lungs, the nose harbors a large range of bacterial species. Many are common to the skin, for example *Staphylococcus, Corynebacterium and Propionibacterium*. In 2017 scientists proved for the first time what had long been suggested — bacteria in the lungs closely resemble the bacterial community in the mouth. Bacteria enter our respiratory tract by microaspiration, they ride in on tiny droplets of saliva from the bacteria-packed mouth.

Many of these bacteria end up at the bottom of the trachea, just where this major airway from the mouth branches off left and right to the lungs. Humans' upright posture and gravity makes this spot a natural landing pad for the inhaled saliva. Coughing sends the collected bacteria and mucus up to the mouth, where they can be expelled from the body. But some bacteria travel all the way to the outermost reaches of the lungs, to the alveoli (tiny air sacs). Here oxygen in the air we breathe diffuses across the epithelial cell membrane of the alveoli into the blood vessels beneath this single cell layer.

Researchers found that wherever the bacteria land, they join a community mostly made up of other newly arrived bacteria. Few bacteria are long-term residents of healthy lungs. Unlike other environments, such as the gut, healthy lungs are inhospitable, with little nutrition and a hypervigilant immune system. They lack the moist, hospitable conditions of the mouth and gut, offering only a thin layer of surfactant to keep the lungs from drying out.

Goblet cells in the trachea and bronchioles trap many bacteria in a mucus before they reach the lungs, while specialized immune cells in the lungs constantly look out for, and destroy, unwelcome bugs. Cilia, the hair-like structures on cells lining the branching bronchioles within the lungs, sweep rhythmically like a biological broom, removing debris and invading microbes.

Scientists think of the lung microbiome as an island where the population of bacteria is determined by the balance between the competing pressures of immigration and elimination.

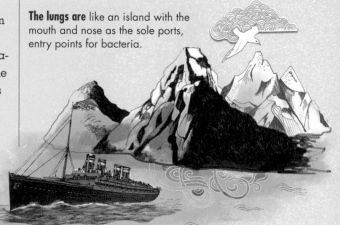

The lungs are like an island with the mouth and nose as the sole ports, entry points for bacteria.

Healthy lungs resemble Antarctica — not quite so cold, perhaps, but overall still an inhospitable environment for bacteria to thrive. A diseased lung is more like a cluster of tropical islands, where patches of inflamed tissue provide a balmy environment for pathogens.

The most common bacteria found in healthy lungs are *Streptococcus*, *Prevotella* and *Veillonella* species, while in diseased lungs bacteria such as *Klebsiella pneumoniae* and *Streptococcus pneumoniae* cause pneumonia, and *Haemophilus influenzae* causes bronchitis.

X-ray shadowing seen in bacterial pneumonia.

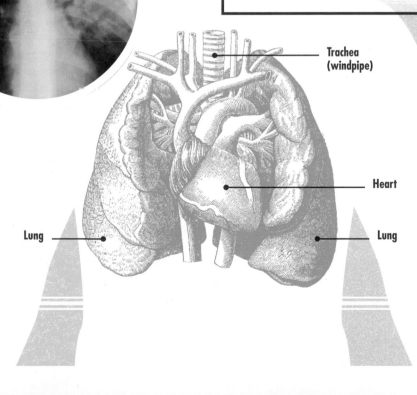

LUNG BACTERIA

Bacteria within the lungs reside within the alveoli. They include:

NORMAL LUNGS:	DISEASED LUNGS:
• *STREPTOCOCCUS SPECIES*	• *STREPTOCOCCUS PNEUMONIAE*
• *PREVOTELLA* SPECIES	• *KLEBSIELLA PNEUMONIAE*
• *VEILLONELLA* SPECIES	• *HAEMOPHILUS INFLUENZAE*
• *PSEUDOMONAS SPECIES*	• *STAPHYLOCOCCUS AUREUS*
• *CORYNEBACTERIUM ACCOLENS*	• *MYCOBACTERIUM TUBERCULOSIS*

Trachea (windpipe)

Heart

Lung

Lung

LUNG BACTERIAL INFECTIONS

Many bacteria lung diseases occur on the back of a viral infection, the most common cause of respiratory tract infections. Viruses, such as the influenza virus damage the single cell epithelial layer. The resulting inflammation allows pathogenic bacteria a chance to multiply and dominate, disrupting the lung microbiome.

Physical factors come into play too — infections and smoking both inhibit the action of the cilia. An inability to cough efficiently (as with the elderly, due to painful back conditions or when asleep) also means that bacteria are not expelled from the lungs; this allows pathogenic bacteria their own breathing space. And coughing at night may not be very efficient when lying horizontal.

Opportunistic bacteria such as *Haemophilus influenzae* (bronchitis) and *Streptococcus pneumoniae* (pneumonia) only cause disease because the lungs' immune system is already compromised.

Some bacteria may also travel in the blood from a "leaky gut." The lungs of very sick patients in intensive care units, such as sufferers of Acute Respiratory Disease Syndrome (ARDS) or sepsis (blood poisoning), carry a disproportionate number of gut bacteria. In these patients antibiotics given for gut infections also help to prevent lung infections. Such diseases are extreme examples, but they demonstrate the consequences of disordered bacterial communities in the gut and lung.

DISTURBING THE EQUILIBRIUM

Some lung diseases are associated with a reduction in bacterial diversity. The chronic bacterial lung infections seen in cystic fibrosis (CF) patients, also associated with disturbed lung microbiomes, provide clues as to what happens in lung infections in general.

The gene defect in CF leads to a build-up of mucus in the body. In the lungs this creates more favorable conditions for bacteria, and particularly for the opportunistic bacteria *Pseudomonas aeruginosa* (see page 75).

Over a decade-long study, researchers found that, as a CF patient's disease progressed, their lung microbiome became less diverse, although the overall numbers of bacteria stayed the same. This was attributed to the regular use of antibiotics, a necessity in CF patients — raising the question of whether there is a tipping point at which antibiotics may do more harm than good. Destroying the pathogenic bacteria is important, but it comes at the cost of losing the good guys too.

Bacteriophages may be the answer. Their name, meaning "eaters of bacteria," says it all — these viruses have shown promise in animal models as effective treatments against chronic *P. aeruginosa* lung infections.

Another study highlights the tropical island effect (see page 92) in one bacteria. In the lungs of CF patients, treatments for *Pseudomonas aeruginosa* infection are sometimes effective in one area, but less so in others. Species of bacteria isolated from each other evolve differently and researchers noted differences in nutritional requirements, the reaction of the immune system and varying antibiotic resistance. Researchers are looking at how regional isolation affects other bacterial lung infections.

Pneumonia can be caused by a virus or a bacteria. The bacteria include *Streptococcus pneumoniae* and *Klebsiella pneumoniae*. When the bacteria infect the lungs, the immune system sends in white blood cells to fight the infection and the alveoli fill with fluid. These clogged-up airways make breathing and efficient gas exchange difficult.

Tuberculosis caused by *Mycobacterium tuberculosis* was once the leading cause of death in the U.S. and Europe, but is now largely a disease of the past. In countries where nutrition is poor and living conditions are crowded, however, or in those whose immune system is compromised (such as AIDS patients), tuberculosis is still a killer, responsible for 1.5 million deaths annually. Multiple rounds of different antibiotics (to minimize resistance) are the preferred treatment, while preventive measures focus on identifying patients, both those with the active disease and carriers who show no signs of infection.

Tuberculosis has been around for at least 20,000 years. However, other lung diseases, such as Legionnaires disease (see page 98), have arisen much more recently.

STREPTOCOCCUS PNEUMONIAE

FIRST DOCUMENTED 1881

GRAM-POSITIVE COCCI

WHAT:
S. pneumoniae is a pathogenic bacterium and a major cause of pneumonia, as the name suggests.

WHERE:
S. pneumoniae causes invasive lung infections by infecting the alveoli. If untreated, it has a high mortality rate of around 30 percent.

HOW:
The bacterium produces a protective capsule that shields it from the immune system in the lung.

CASE NOTES:
S. pneumoniae can become resistant to the antibiotic *penicillin* to a greater or lesser extent, which makes targeting delivery of high concentrations of penicillin a priority.

Streptococcus pneumoniae

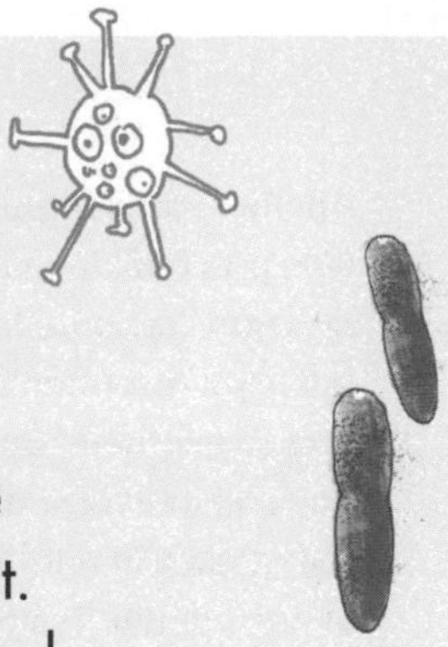

WHAT THE GOOD LUNG BACTERIA DO FOR US

Although lung microbiome studies are 10–15 years behind those of the gut microbiome, there are some fascinating facts to sniff out. Starting with those nasal inhabitants, a bacterium that has attracted attention recently is *Corynebacterium accolens*.

The story of *C. accolens* started in 2011, when it was found that children with high levels of the bacterium in their upper respiratory tract had lower levels of one of the bacteria that causes pneumonia, *Streptococcus pneumoniae*. A chicken and egg scenario perhaps, but in 2016 scientists further showed that *C. accolens* inhibited the growth of *S. pneumoniae* by the action of oleic acid, an antibacterial fatty acid.

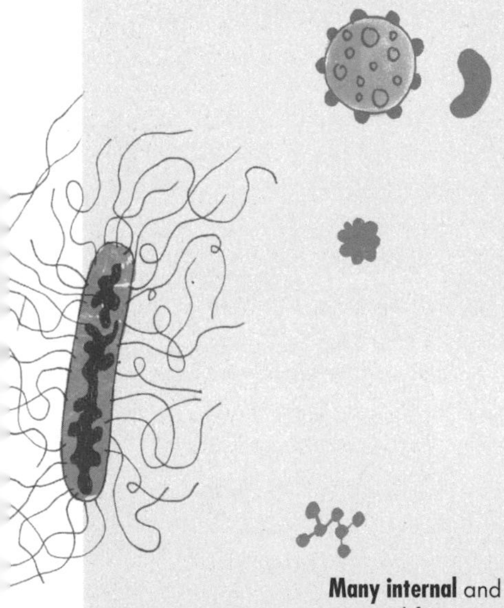

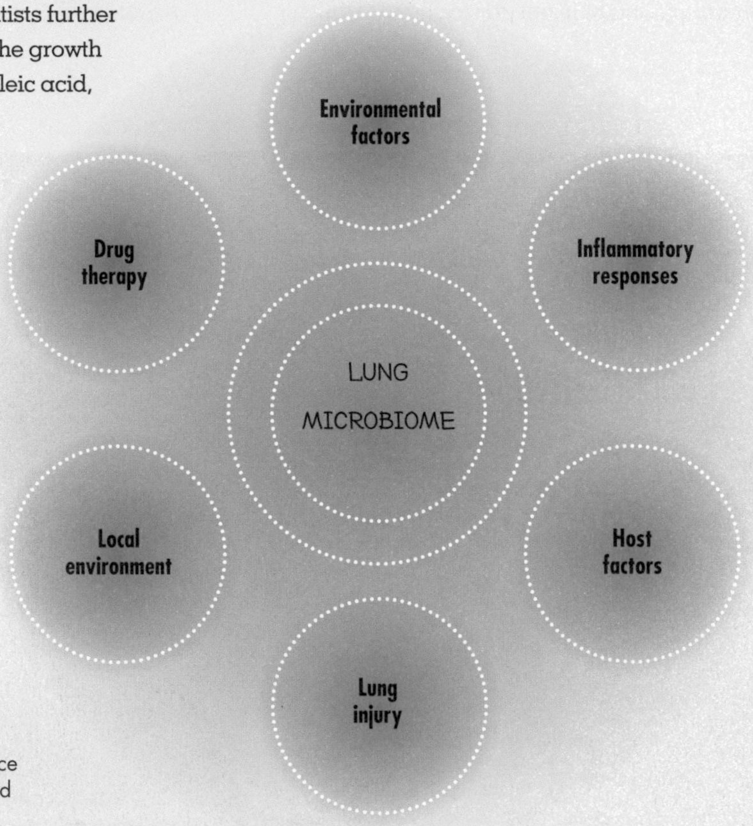

Many internal and external factors influence what bacteria are found in the lung.

Environmental factors

Inflammatory responses

Drug therapy

LUNG MICROBIOME

Host factors

Local environment

Lung injury

CLEANING UP THE HYGIENE HYPOTHESIS

First proposed in 1989, the hygiene hypothesis suggested that we were not being exposed to enough pathogenic microbes — bacteria, viruses and fungi — in our early childhood, and that this was at the heart of the sharp rise in cases of auto-immune diseases (such as multiple sclerosis and Type 1 diabetes) and asthma since the 1950s. Now all the evidence suggests that it is the lack of early exposure to a diverse range of "friendly" bacteria that is important. We need them to train our immune systems to respond appropriately to threats. Without such early training, the body's immune system goes haywire and starts to recognize its own components as foreign, causing the destructive processes seen in autoimmune disease and the inflammation in asthmatic lungs. Birth cohort studies have shown that a deficiency in commensal bacteria in the lungs results in increased sensitivity to allergens. Now scientists are trying to identify which bacteria are important, to develop strategies to help prevent childhood asthma.

HIERARCHY OF HELP

Space and environmental factors are important, as elsewhere in the body. Crowd out the bad guys and make sure the environment remains inhospitable for them. Antibiotic use also reveals the delicate balance required. The administration of a narrow spectrum antibiotic can successfully eradicate chest infections caused by the gram-negative *Haemophilus influenzae*, but leaves untouched the gram-positive *Streptococcus pneumoniae* — which is being kept in check, in part, by the less pathogenic *H. influenzae*. In a vulnerable patient, eradication of the latter suddenly provides a window of opportunity for *S. pneumoniae* to cause havoc, resulting in pneumonia.

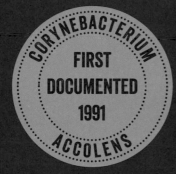

CORYNEBACTERIUM

FIRST DOCUMENTED 1991

ACCOLENS

GRAM-POSITIVE ROD
....

WHAT:
C. accolens is a commensal bacteria of the eyes, ears, nose and throat.

WHERE:
Like *Staphylococcus epidermidis* on the skin, C. accolens exhibits a two-faced approach. In the nose it can have beneficial properties, warding off pathogenic bacteria. Elsewhere it can, in isolated cases, cause a range of infections such as breast abscesses, endocarditis and bone infections.

HOW:
C. accolens seems to switch on its beneficial production of oleic acid, which inhibits pathogens such as *Streptococcus pneumoniae*, when conditions are just right, such as in the nose. Scientists are still researching what makes C. accolens turn into a pathogen elsewhere.

CASE NOTES:
C. accolens is not an easy bacteria to work with. It takes a long time to grow in the laboratory, but scientists are working on a producing a genetically engineered, harmless variant that could prevent pneumnia caused by *S. pneumoniae*.

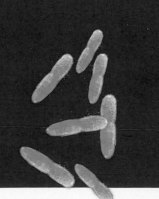

ENCOURAGING THE GOOD AND DISCOURAGING THE BAD

START WITH THE VIRUSES

Many diseases of the lung are caused by viruses. But the damage these cause to the epithelial cell lining often leads to a bacterial infection. So minimizing the chances of getting a viral infection in the first place is important.

Take measures to counteract infections, both viral and bacterial: wash your hands frequently and well, get plenty of sleep, eat a balanced diet and quit smoking. Manage stress to stop the associated hormones from hampering the immune system. Take up any vaccines available, particularly relevant for vulnerable groups such as babies and the elderly, or those with lung diseases such as Chronic Obstructive Pulmonary Disease (COPD). For example, the pneumococcal vaccine protects against pneumonia caused by the bacterium *Streptococcus pneumoniae*.

A LUNG-FRIENDLY DIET

Diet plays a surprising role in lung infections. Obese people are more likely to have respiratory infections, probably because high calorie diets and the resulting obesity disrupt the immune response. Mediterranean diets feature, not only as a healthy way to keep slim, but also for their garlic content. Allicin, a molecule extracted from garlic, has recently been found to be a highly effective killer of an antibiotic-resistant strain of lung bacteria called *Burkholderia cepacia*. You would probably have to eat an uncomfortably large amount of raw garlic to consume enough allicin to be effective, but it may explain why garlic has long been favored for its antibacterial properties.

PROTECTING THE TARGET

Enhancing the action of the lung's epithelial cells is a focus of new preventative therapies for patients prone to diseases such as pneumonia. The epithelial cells are a single cell layer that line the alveoli and facilitate the absorption of oxygen into the blood, but they also double up as the lung's sentinel cells. With an extensive molecular armory at their disposal, these epithelial cells are primed to see off any invading pathogens, or at least to minimize their worst attacks.

A CREATED PROBLEM

In 1973 a group of Scottish tourists returned home from Spain with severe pneumonia. The cause went undiscovered until three years later, when a group of veterans attending the Philadelphia State Convention of the American Legion were similarly afflicted. The mortality rate was 16 percent, sufficiently concerning to warrant detailed investigations, and *Legionella pneumophilia* was discovered. These bacteria are normally only found in fresh water and moist soil, but air-conditioning units, shower heads and whirlpools provide perfect conditions for their growth and distribution. Legionnaire's disease is entirely created. Sanitary regulations now minimize outbreaks, but those that do occur remind us how easy it is for bacteria to gain the upper hand.

One trick is the epithelial cell's ability to secrete an enzyme that opens up the junctions between them. This newly created space allows immune cells to get close to their bacterial target.

Finding ways to control that process is important. High numbers of immune cells, with the resulting inflammation (see page 36), can seriously impede breathing, but too few immune cells means the bacterial infection is not cleared. Another balancing act is required.

New therapies currently in clinical trials include inhibiting the adhesion of virulent pathogens such as *P. aeruginosa* to the epithelial cells and preventing the formation of antibiotic-resistant biofilms. Antibiotic resistance is an increasing problem with bacteria such as *P. aeruginosa* and *S. pneumoniae*, but new methods of delivery such as aerosols fire antibiotics in a concentrated form right to the heart of the action.

Florence Nightingale's recovery "equation": fresh air + friendly bacteria = accelerated recovery from infection.

AN OPEN DOOR (OR WINDOW) APPROACH

When scientists analyzed the airborne microbes that float inside air-conditioned hospital rooms, there was very little overlap with those in the fresh air. Outside the air was full of harmless microbes from plants and soils; inside the numbers were weighted toward harmful viruses and bacteria. Scarce in the outside world, these pathogens had come from the mouths and skin of sick patients.

Florence Nightingale would have had a thing or two to say about that. In the 1850s, during the Crimean War and with no knowledge of the bacterial world, she noticed that patients recovered from infections more quickly when a window was opened. The fresh air brings in harmless environmental bacteria that take up space in our lungs and exclude pathogenic bacteria.

Keeping windows open is not always practical. However, as many of us spend about 90 percent of our time indoors, architects are beginning to design bacteria-friendly buildings. These will help healthy bacteria to get a foothold in our lungs and minimize the available space for the pathogenic kind.

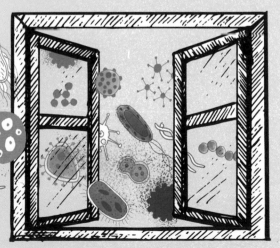

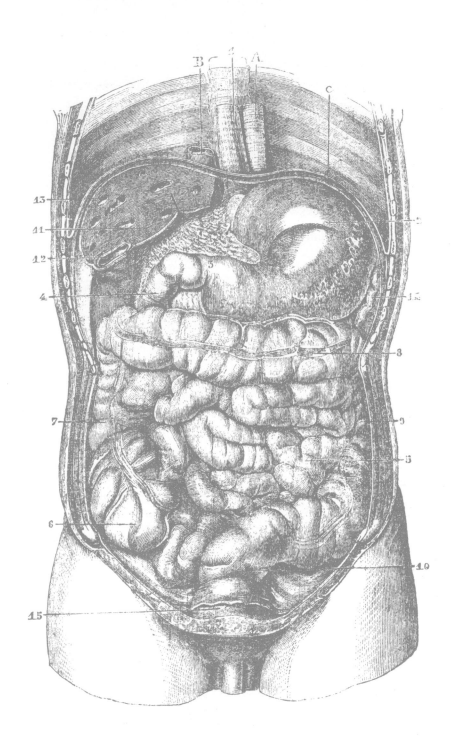

THE GUT

Your gut contains one hundred trillion bacteria, a bacterial load that far exceeds the number of people on the planet and anywhere else on the body. Thankfully these bacteria are mainly a friendly, helpful crowd. Their effects are mind-blowing: from mental health to the immune system, the gut bacteria have a phenomenal influence on our health. The gut is no longer the "forgotten organ."

WHERE AND HOW BACTERIA LIVE IN OUR GUT

The skin is the most obvious barrier with the outside world, while inside the body, curled around neatly beneath the stomach, the gut unravels to provide an even larger area for bacteria to colonize. Each person has their own unique and diverse range of bacteria here, with the numbers of different species sometimes running into the thousands. The challenge is working out which we should be encouraging or discouraging in the quest to keep us healthy and happy.

Some patterns are beginning to emerge. A person's enterotype, the broad profile of their type of gut bacteria, depends on the family of bacteria that dominates in the gut. Regardless of age, gender and ancestry, humans have an enterotype dominated by one of several families of bacteria.

For example, the *Bacteroides* family are experts at breaking down carbohydrates and also have a particular fondness for meat, so are more common in the guts of people who are love burgers and sausages. *Bacteroides* are known for their tidy nature so they work best alongside other bacteria that live off the numerous waste products floating in the gut. In contrast, *Prevotella* bacteria dominate in the guts of vegetarians and, like many bacteria, are involved in the production of vitamins.

Bacteria arrive in our body every time we eat, and diet is the biggest driver of our gut enterotype. Food passes down the esophagus into the stomach, where the main process of digestion begins. Beyond that, in the small intestine, the digested carbohydrates, proteins and fats are absorbed into the bloodstream. The peristalsis of the gut (involuntary rhythmic muscular movements) pushes the food along the digestive tract, and the highly acid conditions of the stomach and the small intestine are inhospitable environments for bacteria. So although these areas are certainly not sterile, they contain relatively small numbers of bacteria in healthy subjects.

Beyond the small intestine, any undigested material (mainly fiber) carries on to the large intestine, where the food spends the longest time — up to 16 hours. This means that in the large intestine (the colon) the bacterial concentration and variety increases dramatically. Anaerobic bacteria outnumber aerobic bacteria here by a factor of between 100 and 1,000 to one, reflecting the ability of anaerobic bacteria to adapt to the hostile low oxygen environment.

At any given point in the gut there is variation, with distinct bacterial communities forming in microhabitats, such as the gut lumen (the space in which the food moves along), crypts (glands) in both the small and large intestine and the colon mucus layers. These crypts and the mucus layers are important as they provide a reservoir of bacteria to repopulate the lumen after an infection.

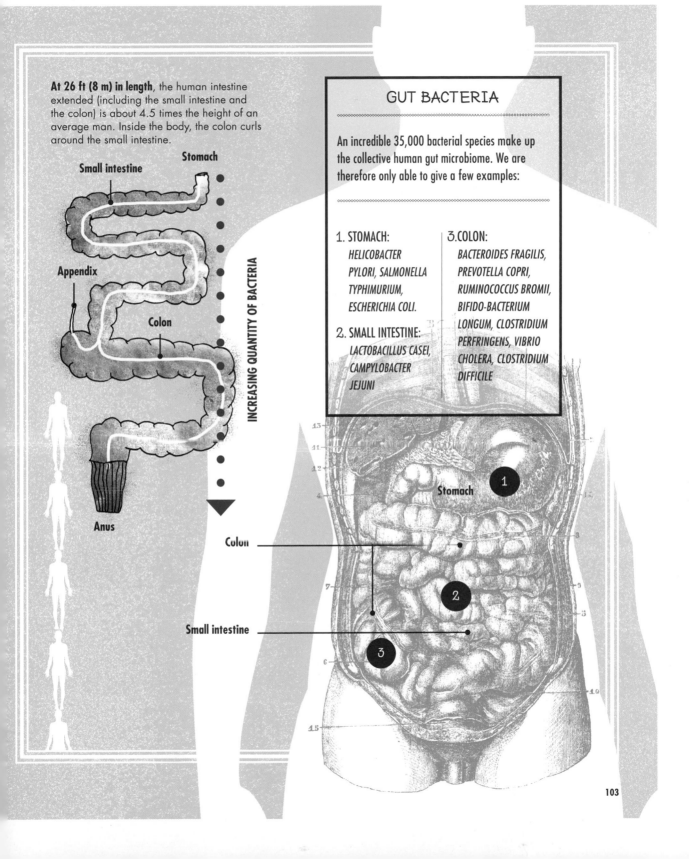

At 26 ft (8 m) in length, the human intestine extended (including the small intestine and the colon) is about 4.5 times the height of an average man. Inside the body, the colon curls around the small intestine.

Stomach

Small intestine

Appendix

Colon

Anus

INCREASING QUANTITY OF BACTERIA

GUT BACTERIA

An incredible 35,000 bacterial species make up the collective human gut microbiome. We are therefore only able to give a few examples:

1. STOMACH:
   HELICOBACTER PYLORI, SALMONELLA TYPHIMURIUM, ESCHERICHIA COLI.

2. SMALL INTESTINE:
   LACTOBACILLUS CASEI, CAMPYLOBACTER JEJUNI

3. COLON:
   BACTEROIDES FRAGILIS, PREVOTELLA COPRI, RUMINOCOCCUS BROMII, BIFIDO-BACTERIUM LONGUM, CLOSTRIDIUM PERFRINGENS, VIBRIO CHOLERA, CLOSTRIDIUM DIFFICILE

Stomach

Colon

Small intestine

GUT BACTERIAL INFECTIONS

Some gut diseases have a well-characterized single bacterial cause that enters the body via the gut and produces significant symptoms there, and frequently elsewhere too. Contaminated food or water are the most common sources of a gut bacterial infection.

Tummy trouble, in the form of food poisoning, is caused by bacteria such as *Campylobacter*, *Salmonella*, *E. coli* and *Listeria* (see page 130). But other types of bacterial infections, such as the more tropical diseases cholera and typhoid, or an imbalance of gut bacteria must be considered too.

Scientists have certainly identified some long-term residents in the gut that can lead to disease. *Helicobacter pylori*, for example, is found in the stomach of about 40 percent of the population, most of the time without problems, but in about 15 percent of people it can cause ulcers. Dr. Barry Marshall first proved it could be a pathogen when, in 1984, he swallowed a vial of *H. pylori*. Not to be tried at home! However, it did result in a 2005 Nobel Prize for Dr. Marshall and colleague Dr. Robin Warren. *H. pylori* infections have also been associated with an increased risk of stomach cancer.

VACCINATION SUCCESSES

Vaccines for gut bacterial infections include cholera and typhoid. Prevalent in developing countries, typhoid fever is contracted from food or water contaminated with infected feces or urine. Caused by a bacterium called *Salmonella typhi*, which is related to the bacteria that cause salmonella food poisoning, typhoid can spread beyond the gut, affecting many organs. Without prompt treatment, it can lead to serious complications and may be fatal.

IRRITABLE BOWEL SYNDROME (IBS)

Symptoms of IBS include stomach cramps and bloating, alongside a change in bowel habits and sometimes depression and anxiety. The causes are likely to involve a number of factors, but our gut bacteria are certainly implicated, and sufferers will know that periods of stress can make IBS worse. Experiments on mice suggest that the gut bacteria/brain connection is behind this, alongside an unbalanced gut bacteria profile. Understanding why harmful gut bacteria numbers are higher in IBS patients is critical to understanding the condition. The modulation of gut bacteria seems to be the way forward, following the idea that expansion of beneficial bacterial species (*Lactobacilli* and *Bifidobacteria*) and the reduction of harmful bacteria (*Clostridium*, *E. coli*, *Salmonella*, *Shigella* and *Pseudomonas*) should alleviate IBS symptoms, both physical and mental.

ESCHERICHIA COLI

FIRST DOCUMENTED 1885

GRAM-NEGATIVE ROD

Antibiotics are used for most *E. coli* infections, except in the case of *E. coli 0157* where they can aggravate symptoms and increase the chance of developing a more severe illness known as hemolytic-uremic syndrome. *E. coli* bacteria can also cause infections outside the intestine if it is torn or damaged, for example by an injury or a disease such as inflammatory bowel disease (IBD).

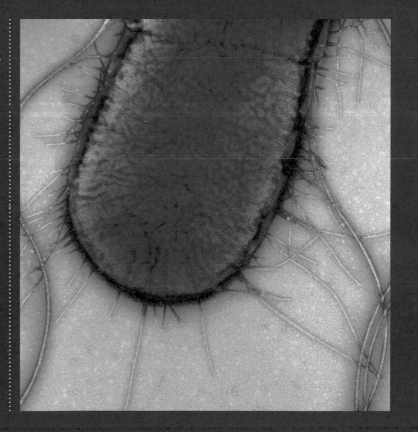

Escherichia coli showing the flagellum used for movement.

WHAT:
Escherichia coli is a commensal gut bacteria. Most strains are harmless but some can cause disease, including urinary tract infections and food poisoning.

WHERE:
The incubation period for food poisoning caused by *E. coli* is typically one to eight days. The symptoms of cramps and diarrhea usually last for a few days to a week.

HOW:
Most cases of *E. coli* food poisoning from the 0157 strain, which produces a toxin known as Shiga toxin, occur after eating undercooked beef (particularly ground beef) or drinking unpasteurized milk.

VIBRIO

FIRST DOCUMENTED 1883

CHOLERA

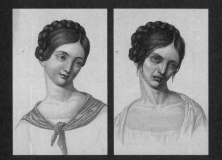

An 1830s engraving showing a Viennese woman, before contracting cholera and in the later stages of the disease. Her face bears the blue tinge of severe dehydration.

GRAM-NEGATIVE CURVED ROD

WHAT
A water-dwelling bacterium.

WHERE:
V. cholera enters the body via the mouth, usually in contaminated water or food, and sets up an infection in the small intestine.

HOW:
V. cholera infections cause diarrhea and vomiting. In severe cases death can occur from circulatory failure or multiple organ failure.

CASE NOTES:
Cholera was thought to be an airborne disease until 1854, when Dr. John Snow identified a contaminated water pump as the source of a cholera outbreak in London. His "germ" theory of disease was not accepted until the 1860s. Today cholera causes an estimated 120,000 deaths per year and is prevalent in some 80 countries. Food and water hygiene precautions are usually enough to prevent infection, but a vaccine is available for aid workers where there is a cholera outbreak.

Light micrograph (photo taken through a microscope) of *Vibrio cholera*.

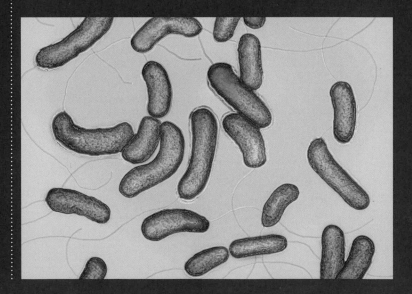

DYSBIOSIS AND DISEASE

Many diseases do not appear to be linked to any single species of bacteria, but rather to dysbiosis, a disruption in the balance of the gut bacteria. This disruption can have a number of causes, such as antibiotic treatment for an infection, a dramatic change in lifestyle, such as a rather indulgent weekend, or a bout of food poisoning.

Chronic bowel diseases, such as the inflammatory bowel diseases (ulcerative colitis and Crohn's disease) and IBS, seem to be the result of complicated interactions between the gut microbiome and immune system. Celiac disease is an autoimmune disease of the gut which, like other autoimmune diseases including rheumatoid arthritis and multiple sclerosis, may be triggered by a bacterial infection in the gut. Connections between the gut bacteria and diseases such as diabetes, carcinoma and HIV are also now being explored.

The gut "garden" relies on a healthy "cross-pollination" between gut cells, the immune system and bacterial species to maintain a bacterial diversity and homeostasis.

TREATMENT

Although the connections between gut bacteria and different diseases are still being made, the hope is that this research will lead to new treatments. The huge problem of antibiotic resistance (see page 47) and the associated issue of the sledgehammer approach of antibiotics mean that as work to discover and develop new antibiotics continues, other more holistic methods are also being investigated. Encouraging the growth of good bacteria using prebiotics and probiotics (see pages 160–61), and transferring good bacteria from healthy people to the unwell (see page 163) are all being explored as treatments. In diseases such as colitis, caused by bacterial overgrowth, researchers are looking at how they can hijack the body's existing systems for controlling bacterial growth — namely, small pieces of genomic material known as micro RNA. Such material is produced by gut cells, which pass through bacterial cell walls and affect their growth. Manipulating the microbiome for better health is now receiving a great deal of attention in the scientific community.

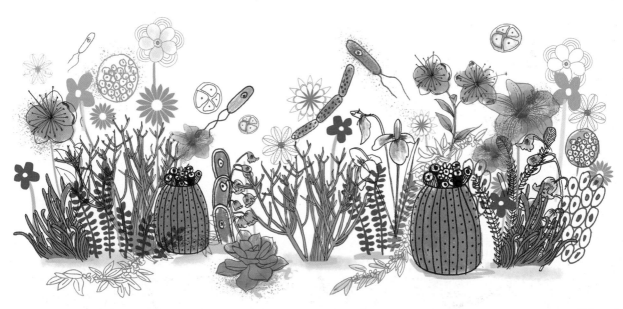

WHAT THE GOOD GUT BACTERIA DO FOR US

The bacteria in our large intestine work hard to keep us healthy. They get actively involved in our metabolism, control our immune responses, prevent the colonization of pathogens and stimulate the immune system, to name a few of their roles.

Gut bacteria play a central role, influencing many different areas of the body, as shown here.

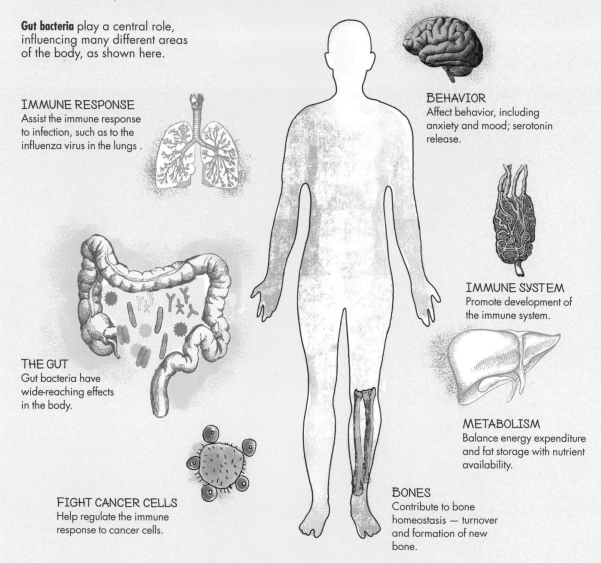

IMMUNE RESPONSE
Assist the immune response to infection, such as to the influenza virus in the lungs.

BEHAVIOR
Affect behavior, including anxiety and mood; serotonin release.

IMMUNE SYSTEM
Promote development of the immune system.

THE GUT
Gut bacteria have wide-reaching effects in the body.

METABOLISM
Balance energy expenditure and fat storage with nutrient availability.

FIGHT CANCER CELLS
Help regulate the immune response to cancer cells.

BONES
Contribute to bone homeostasis — turnover and formation of new bone.

SHORT-CHAIN FATTY ACIDS

Your friendly gut bacteria produce short-chain fatty acids as part of the fermentation of fiber. These fatty acids are the primary energy source for the cells in your gut. They do more than just nourish your cells, however — acetic acid is vital to muscle health, while propionic acid helps your body tissues to respond to insulin, protecting against metabolic diseases such as diabetes. Butyric acid helps to keep the immune system in check and acts as an anti-inflammatory.

Happily, the more fiber you digest, the more fiber-fermenting bacteria, such as *Bifidobacteria*, you will be able to support in your gut. The more of these bacteria in your gut, the more beneficial short-chain fatty acids will be produced.

VITAMINS

It may be a surprise to learn that essential vitamins are not always derived from our diet. Some can be made by our gut bacteria. The magnitude of this contribution is currently poorly understood, although it is estimated that up to half of our Vitamin K daily requirement (which helps blood to clot and wounds to heal) is produced by gut bacteria. Complex chemical reactions are involved. For example, Vitamin B_{12} is pieced together as an elaborate molecular jigsaw involving around 30 individual components; a B_{12} deficiency produces a lack of energy and tiredness. The assembly of Vitamin B_{12} can be carried out by at least 20 bacteria in the large intestine, including *Pseudomonas denitrificans*. Other vitamins such as Vitamin B_1 (thiamine) and Vitamin B_2 (riboflavin), which help to boost energy, are found in unprocessed plant and animal products, but can also be produced by bacteria in the colon. Vitamin B_1 contains sulfur; it is responsible for that bad egg smell associated with people whose enterotype is dominated by *Prevotella* bacteria.

BACTERIA AND WEIGHT

Germ-free mice, bred and housed in sterile conditions, reveal a great deal about obesity. These mice eat more than their littermates and take longer to digest their food; their immune systems are also compromised. If scientists give these mice gut bacteria from obese humans, they are more likely to gain weight than if they receive bacteria from non-obese people. Gut bacteria seem to regulate how efficiently we process food.

Studies in humans have shown that the guts of some obese people have less bacterial diversity and more bacteria that can break down carbohydrates compared with those who are slim. These obese individuals are more efficient at extracting every last morsel of nutrient from food and therefore gain weigh more easily — a useful asset in a famine, but not in a feast.

Low levels of bacterial infections may also play a role. These do not produce any obvious symptoms, but show up with raised levels of inflammatory markers in the blood. Signaling molecules that are produced by bacteria can lock onto organs such as the liver and encourage the deposition of fat.

Another theory is that gut bacteria are responsible for cravings for chocolate. Bacteria can produce molecules small enough to travel across the blood vessels into the brain (see pages 152–53). The idea is that the bacteria "reward" us when we provide the delicious — and to them, nutritious — chocolate bar, by sending neurotransmitters to the brain that light up our pleasure receptors.

INFLUENCING THE EFFECT OF MEDICINES

Our gut bacteria influence how we metabolize medicines, probably to a much larger extent than we currently realize. For example, paracetamol can be more toxic for some people than others — some gut bacteria produce a substance that influences the liver's ability to process the drug.

Cancer patients respond best to treatments when they have the right mix of bacteria in their guts — which may be one reason why success rates in chemotherapy regimens are lower than we would wish. Avoiding antibiotics while having chemo-therapy is part of the story, potentially boosting the number who respond to treatment by 40 percent. Antibiotics are often life-saving drugs, but their use has a price — disruption to the delicate balance in the gut bacteria.

Profiling a patient's gut microbiome, and person-alizing therapies accordingly, is right up there with genetic profiling as a way of fine-tuning treatments for intractable diseases such as cancer.

CONTROL OF IMMUNE RESPONSES

As in other areas of the body, many gut bacteria protect us simply by occupying the space that would otherwise be taken by a pathogenic bacteria. Unlike the skin, which has three layers, in the gut just a single layer of epithelial cells separates what passes through the gut lumen from the blood that circulates around the body. Immune surveillance is therefore a critical function of the gut lining, which detects and reacts to the molecules and bacteria carried through the gut.

The education and regulation of the immune response is one of the many hats our gut bacteria wear. Helpful bacteria assist us to distinguish friend from foe — the key aim of the immune system (see pages 34–37). In the gut, the large intestine, which contains regular deposits of immune cells, is the center of this activity. Here the immune system is highly reactive — interactions of commensal bacteria with the immune cell centers stimulate the production of antibodies (immunoglobulin A), cytokines (immunoregulatory molecules) and regulatory T cells. These bacterial/immune system interactions modulate our response to pathogens and may be part of the trigger and/or regulation of autoimmune diseases — for instance rheumatoid arthritis and multiple sclerosis (MS).

KEEPING US HAPPY?

No system in the body works in isolation, and nowhere is this more obvious than the pivotal role played by gut bacteria. It is now known that there is a great deal of cross talk between the central nervous system, including the brain, the localized nerves in the gut and gut bacteria. Known as the gut–brain axis (see pages 152–53), this two-way communication system can influence our moods as well as our health.

That sinking feeling in your stomach before an exam is all part of this two-way interaction. Studies in mice and preliminary results in humans have shown that our gut bacteria can influence not only physical diseases such as IBS and diabetes, but also potentially our emotions (see pages 150–51) and our responses to stress and pain.

These studies are difficult to conduct as it is unlikely that a single bacterium is involved; deter-mining precisely which bacteria to encourage is not straightforward. In addition, how people feel is often highly subjective and open to misinterpretation. Nev-ertheless, the idea that we can manipulate emotions using our gut bacteria is an intriguing prospect and one that requires some serious input — both in terms of research and dietary changes.

BACTEROIDES

FIRST DOCUMENTED 1898

FRAGILIS

GRAM-NEGATIVE ROD

WHAT:
A commensal bacteria in the large intestine.

HOW:
Having B. fragilis on board is generally a good thing. When fed to mice it helped restore their T cells to normal levels. This effect could be achieved with just a single molecule, called PSA, found on the bacteria's cell surface. Administration of PSA to mice could prevent and cure inflammatory diseases such as colitis and multiple sclerosis.

WHERE:
B. fragilis is a normal inhabitant of the colon, but can cause infections if it escapes into the bloodstream or surrounding tissue after surgery or other infections.

CASE NOTES:
This is a keeper but it should come with a health warning. Much of the research on its remarkable properties has only been done in mice and it remains to be seen whether such stellar results are observed in humans.

Bacteroides fragilis

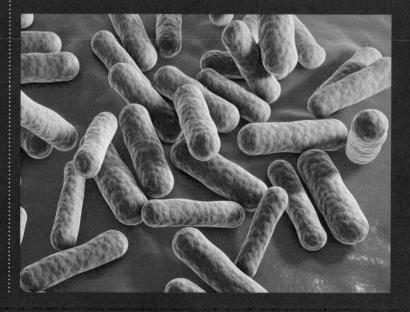

ENCOURAGING THE GOOD AND DISCOURAGING THE BAD

There is a highly complex series of interactions between our brain, our other organ systems, the bacteria in our gut and the food that we eat, all with an underlying genetic influence. We cannot easily manipulate the function of our brain or our genetic profiles, but we can alter our diets.

As we have seen with obese individuals, there may be more to gaining weight than just eating the wrong sort of food. Our gut bacteria have a pivotal role to play, such that our diets may also regulate all sorts of diseases. These range from chronic diseases that directly affect the gut, such as Crohn's disease, to those that affect other areas of the body, such as rheumatoid arthritis.

Eating the wrong food could make your gut bacteria see red.

GUT-HEALTHY FOODS

You can help to create a healthy and diverse community of bacteria in your gut by eating a varied diet that includes the following:

- Plenty of vegetables and fruit. Remember that the less processed they are, the more fiber they have

- Foods rich in antioxidants, such as pecans, blueberries and chocolate to promote diversity in the gut microbiome

- Healthy fats, such as those found in avocados and walnuts. This is another good source of energy for some of your friendly gut bacteria

- Good quality protein, such as fish, eggs and minimally processed meat, as a source of amino acids for the amino acid-fermenting bacteria in your gut — as opposed to meats containing additives, such as bacon or the meat in hot dogs

- Foods rich in healthy bacteria, including probiotic fermented foods such as yogurt with live cultures (see pages 160–61), to help encourage their colonization in your gut

- Restrict consumption of refined carbohydrates and sugars. Most are absorbed before they reach your gut bacteria, so do not provide the bacteria with any nourishment

A GUT-FRIENDLY DIET

It is well known that eating a Mediterranean-style diet (lots of colorful vegetables and fruit, fish, pulses, nuts, olive oil, along with small amounts of red meat, dairy, red wine and very little processed or high sugar foods) benefits your physical health. Not only are these foods good for your heart, skin and bone health, but they are also all foods that friendly gut bacteria love. By eating these foods, we encourage bacteria that regulate our immune system and produce vital vitamins, neurotransmitters and "happy" hormones such as serotonin and dopamine. The prominent role for the gut–brain axis means that your diet might also influence your emotions, anxiety and levels of depression (see pages 150–51).

DITCH THE SALT

Salt could be related to high blood pressure because of its effect on gut bacteria. A recent study found that mice fed a high-salt diet had a reduction of good gut bacteria such as *Lactobacillus* and an increased production of immune cells linked to high blood pressure. Feeding the salty mice with the lost bacteria reversed the effect, and early data from a human study has supported this. Regulating the gut bacteria that link salt intake and heart health may be one way forward in the fight against high blood pressure and heart disease.

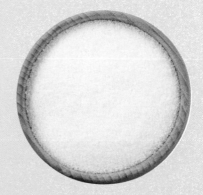

A DIET FOR LIFE

Our diet governs our gut bacteria from day one (see pages 134–35), so maintaining a healthy diet is likely to be important throughout our lives.

A recent study suggested that we might need to pay more attention to the gut bacteria profile of our increasingly elderly population. Those in long-term residential care had significantly less diverse gut bacteria than those living in the community, and this lower diversity was associated with frailty and ill health. Finding ways to manipulate our gut bacteria later in life, through dietary changes and otherwise, may decrease the number of twilight years spent in ill health.

THE BIOTICS

Antibiotics are important tools in our anti-pathogen toolbox, but overuse is causing problems in the gut. Antibiotics change our gut bacteria, unfortunately wiping out the good as well as the bad. Although bacterial communities largely bounce back,

Keeping food chilled minimizes the growth of pathogenic bacteria.

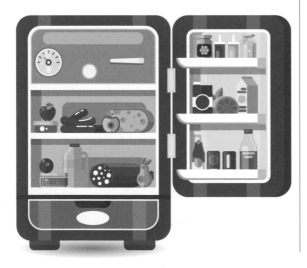

THE FOUR Cs

Contaminated food is the main way we pick up gut bacteria that cause food poisoning. Food standards agencies recommend some simple but effective measures to avoid these: cleaning, cooking, chilling and avoiding cross-contamination.

Storage instructions and sell-by dates are helpful too; relying on appearance and smell alone is not enough.

frequent rounds of antibiotics dent the gut's long-term diversity. And when the barrier of a diverse bacterial community disappears the gut becomes "porous," enabling opportunistic pathogens such as *Salmonella typhi* and *Clostridium difficile* to exploit any uneaten nutrients and colonize any available space.

Another approach is to add beneficial bacteria in the form of probiotics (see pages 160–61). The use of probiotics, even if you have not taken any antibiotics, is likely to be helpful in ensuring a healthy population of gut bacteria. Much research is still needed on how to get enough of the right bacteria into our guts, but the early results from the use of probiotics in diseases such as inflammatory bowel disease (IBD) are encouraging. Help might also be at hand from prebiotics, which can selectively nourish beneficial bacteria (see pages 160–61).

Vegetables contain high quantities of plant fiber that cannot be digested by humans, but they feed our gut bacteria as prebiotics.

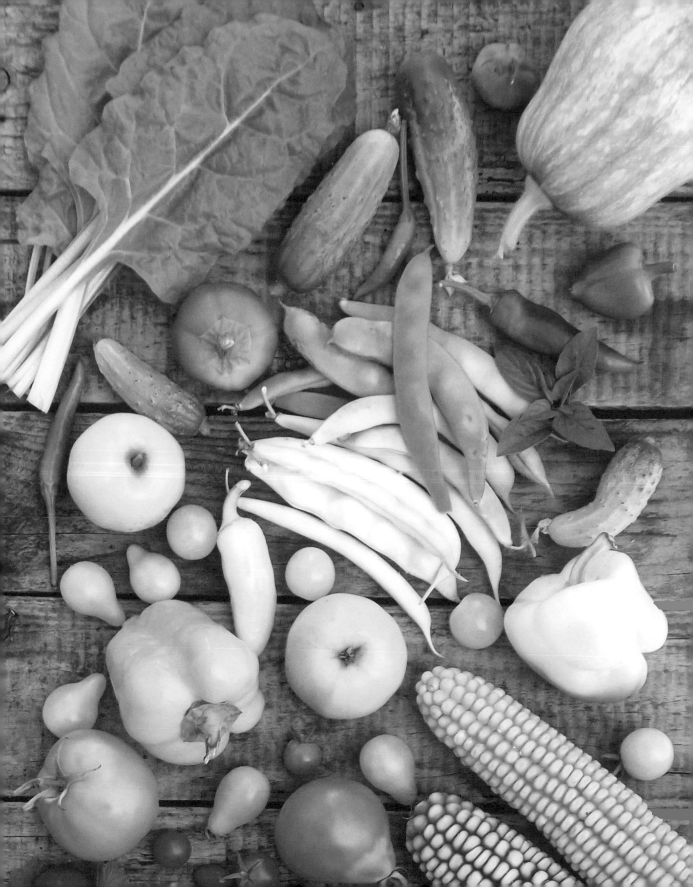

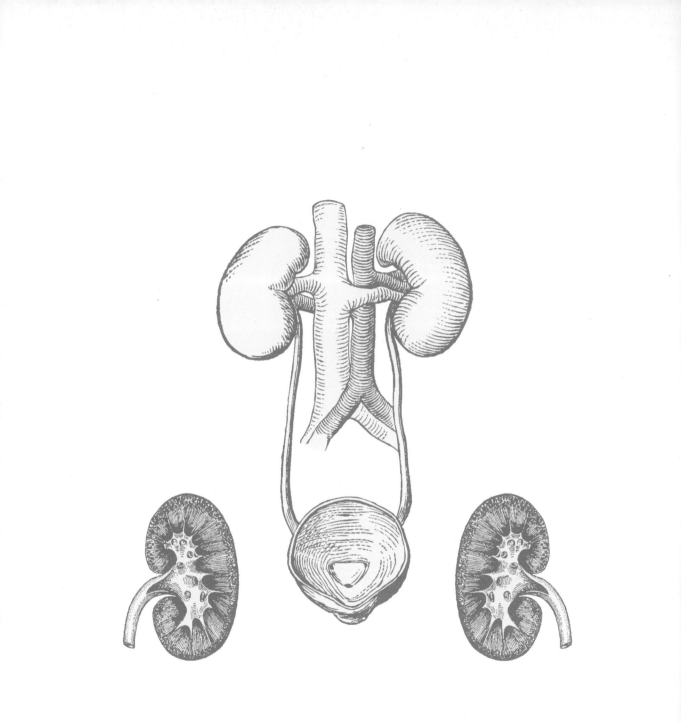

THE UROGENITAL SYSTEM

The composition of the bacteria in these sensitive areas is vital for health. Of all the sites analyzed in the Human Microbiome Project, the vagina has the lowest bacterial diversity. However, low diversity is normal here and high diversity is associated with disease. In men, some bacteria on the penis have recently been added to the list of risk factors for HIV infections.

WHERE AND HOW BACTERIA LIVE IN OUR UROGENITAL SYSTEM

In women, bacteria have been detected in the cervix, fallopian tubes and uterus (womb). However, like those in other "hidden" areas of the body, they have only recently revealed themselves and no-one is quite sure of their function — at least not in a baby-free uterus.

More commonly, bacteria set up camp in the vagina. Here they protect against pathogenic bacteria and fungal infections, partly by colonizing the available space. Vaginal bacteria actively help to decrease the pH inside the vagina, making it harder for other, less acid-loving bacteria to get a look in. The acidic mucus secreted in the vaginal walls also wards off these bacteria.

A bacteria profile can vary widely between individual women. The latest research suggests that there is no "normal" set of bacteria in the vagina: each woman has her own healthy state. Major factors influencing this are ethnicity, sexual activity and a woman's hormonal state (at puberty/menstruating/pregnant/pre- or post-menopausal).

Women fall into one of five categories in terms of their vaginal bacteria profile. Four of these groups are dominated by lactic acid-producing *Lactobacillus* species. These species (*L. crispatus*, *L. iners*, *L. gasseri* and *L. jensenii*) seem to be specific to the human vagina. The fifth group have predominantly anaerobic bacteria (such as *Pseudomonas* and *Acinetobacter*), possibly associated with increased susceptibility to infections.

What happens in the vagina influences what goes on deeper inside the rest of the reproductive tract. The proportion of *Lactobacillus* reduces in these areas gradually, but in the uterus it is still in the region of 30 percent (see opposite).

In men, the penis is home to a variety of bacteria, both in the urethra and on the foreskin. These are influenced by a man's age, sexual activities and whether or not he is circumcised. Compared with the gut, mouth or vagina, there are far fewer bacteria in total in or on the penis, but, not surprisingly, these are shared with sexual partners. This is particularly the case with those more prevalent in women with vaginosis, such as the *Gardnerella vaginalis*, *Atopobium vaginae*, *Megasphaera* and *Prevotella* species, which are transferred from the penis to the vagina. *Lactobacillus* is not a common finding on the penis, but is one of the most common bacteria found in the urethra in healthy men.

The bacterial population of the female urogenital system is primarily a story of the dominant *Lactobacillus* species.

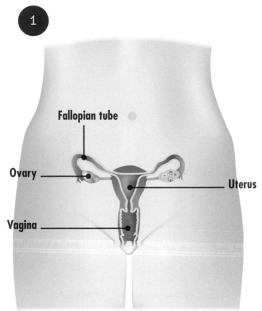

Fallopian tube

Ovary

Vagina

Uterus

UROGENITAL BACTERIA

The bacteria associated with the human reproductive and urinary systems include the following:

1. FEMALE

VAGINA: 90% Lactobacillus species, Chlamydia trachomatis, Gonorrhea neisseria

UTERUS: 30% Lactobacillus species

FALLOPIAN TUBE: 1% Lactobacillus species

URETHRA: Escherichia coli

2. MALE

PENIS: Gardnerella vaginalis, Atropobium vaginae, Chlamydia trachomatis, Megasphaera and Prevotella species

URETHRA: Lactobacillus, Streptococcus, Prevotella and Fusobacterium species.

Lactobacillus **features** in the male urogenital system too, but usually only in the uretha. The penis is home to a variety of bacteria.

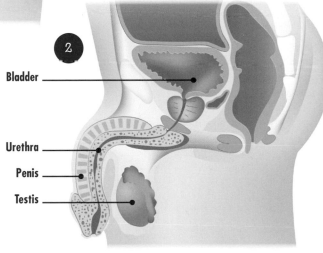

Bladder

Urethra

Penis

Testis

THE FAMILY JEWELS

Like the eye and the brain, the testes are an immune-privileged site, where the body tolerates foreign material without producing an inflammatory reaction. This was once thought to be because sites like the testes were "hidden" from the immune system. Now it is known to be a combination of physical structures, specialized cells and the immune system working to keep the testes free from infection.

UROGENITAL TRACT

It is not just the skin that envelops the penis that is inhabited by bacteria. Scientists have begun to identify bacteria that live in the urogenital tract, a site that was once considered sterile in the absence of infection. Some men pass urine containing a variety of *Lactobacilli* and *Streptococcus* species, whereas others contain more anaerobic bacteria like *Prevotella* and *Fusobacterium*. There is no standout formula for a healthy urogenital tract and, like the penis, it remains an understudied area of the body.

The story in women is similar and, with up to 20 percent of the world's women suffering from urinary tract infections at any one time, the need to understand the normal bacteria and their role in the urogenital tract is now pressing.

The urinary tract is resistant to bacterial colonization, despite frequent contamination with colonic bacteria. Frequent emptying of the bladder flushes out bacteria, while various immunological mechanisms and mucosal barriers help prevent bacterial infections from taking hold inside the urethra. The bladder does not provide much of a meal for bacteria so, in order to survive and grow, pathogens like *E. coli* (see page 105) produce enzymes and toxins that damage the bladder to release nutrients.

E. coli causes more than 75 percent of urinary tract infections. In these bacteria-infected human epithelial cells, the cultures are stained to show the cell nuclei (blue), *E. coli Shiga* toxin (red) and the epithelial cells (green).

SEXUALLY TRANSMITTED AND URINARY TRACT BACTERIAL INFECTIONS

Sharing bacteria is a perennial issue, both from sexual activity and "contamination" from the nearby bowel.

A WORLDWIDE PROBLEM

Sexually transmitted diseases (STDs) have a profound impact on sexual and reproductive health worldwide. Three bacteria between them cause over 200 million new infections annually: chlamydia (131 million), gonorrhea (78 million) and syphilis (7.6 million). The good news is that all of these are curable with antibiotics, unlike the viral STD.

Some STDs have serious consequences beyond the immediate impact of the infection itself. For example, pelvic inflammatory disease, which can have long-term effects on fertility in women, is an infection caused by bacteria. In around one in four cases, it is sexually transmitted by a bacterium such as Chlamydia trachomatis or Neisseria gonorrheae, when these bacteria travel from the vagina to the uterus, fallopian tubes and/or ovaries. And mother-to-child transmission of an STD such as syphilis can result in premature birth, congenital deformities or stillbirth.

THE "SOCIAL" DISEASES

STDs, also euphemistically known as "social diseases," are infections transmitted during sexual contact. As many of these bacterial infections are symptomless, bacteria can be spread by one person to another with the former unaware that they have been infected.

Like chlamydia and syphilis, gonorrhea is often an asymptomatic bacterial infection; it can remain undiagnosed in up to 90 percent of men. Gonorrhea is caused by Neisseria gonorrhoeae bacteria and, like chlamydia, can cause urethritis. This leads to burning or pain on urination and discharge from the urethra in men or the vagina in women.

Syphilis may have been bought back from the Americas by Christopher Columbus. It is certainly known to have ravaged Europe in the late 15th/early 16th centuries when it became known as "the great pox." The side effects of early treatments, such as mercury and the arsenic-based drug Salvarsan, were often so severe that they themselves led to premature death. With the advent of penicillin, infection rates plummeted. Today syphilis is most commonly found in sub-Saharan Africa, where it is associated with other STDs such as HIV/AIDS.

Syphilis is a bacterial infection caused by the Treponema pallidum bacteria. It is treatable with antibiotics when the first signs of an ulcer appear on the genitals. If left untreated other organs can become involved, however, leading to unsightly skin rashes, arthritis, kidney problems and even brain infections in later years.

CHLAMYDIA

FIRST DOCUMENTED 1907

TRACHOMATIS

GRAM-NEGATIVE COCCI

CASE NOTES:
C. trachomatis is often a "silent" infection in the urogenital regions. Around 75 percent of women and 50 percent of men who are infected show no symptoms. That's not great news, as untreated infections can result in serious complications such as pelvic inflammatory disease, infertility and ectopic pregnancies in women. Inflammation in the testicles can also lead to infertility in men. It is all about not acquiring the unwanted bacteria in the first place. Prevention is recommended in the form of counseling or behavioral approaches, or barrier methods such as condoms. Thankfully you can be tested for *C. trachomatis* whether you show symptoms or not and antibiotic treatment is usually successful.

WHAT:
C. trachomatis is the bacteria that causes the majority of reported sexually transmitted diseases worldwide. In the developing world the eye disease trachoma is endemic (see page 74).

ing the bacteria's potential effects on the body. Symptoms in both sexes can include a genital discharge, genital itching/inflammation and painful urination.

A cell infected with ***Chlamydia trachomatis*** (blue); the cell's nucleus is colored purple.

WHERE:
C. trachomatis infects the epithelial cell layer of the cervix, urethra and rectum through sexual contact; another strain infects non-genital sites such as the lungs and eyes.

HOW:
Chlamydia comes from the Greek words "chlamys," meaning cloak, reflecting the bacteria's ability to protect itself from the actions of the immune system, and "trachomatis," meaning rough or harsh, highlight-

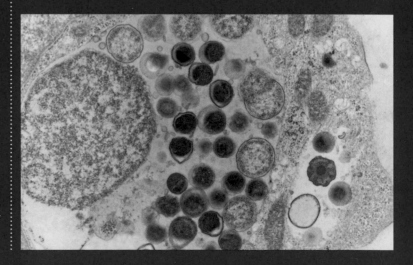

WOMEN-ONLY

A high diversity of vaginal bacteria and a lack of *Lactobacillus* species is associated with vaginosis, the most prevalent cause of abnormal vaginal discharge in women of childbearing age. Those most severely affected experience an offensive, fishy-smelling discharge that recurs frequently, often around the time of menstruation. Others may have vaginosis transiently and asymptomatically. It usually responds to treatment with antibiotics, but can relapse rapidly and is a risk factor for problems in pregnancy such as late miscarriages and premature birth.

MEN-ONLY

When the mechanisms that preserve the immune-privileged state of the testes are disrupted, infections with bacteria cause orchitis, an inflammation and swelling of the testes, which can affect fertility. Some bacteria, such as *C. trachomatis*, can also infect the end of the penis, the glans, causing redness and irritation.

HONEYMOON DISEASE

Women have drawn the short straw with urinary tract infections (UTIs), literally. The urethra is significantly shorter in women compared with men — 2in (4cm) versus 8in (20cm) — so bacteria from the outside can easily reach the female bladder. Among adults aged 20–50 years, UTIs are 50 times more common in women. *Escherichia coli* (see page 105) is the cause of 75 percent of UTIs.

Bacteria can be transferred directly from the anus or through sexual contact, hence the name "honeymoon" disease, for some cases of cystitis. Urinary tract infections occur when the bacteria ascend the urethra to the bladder and sometimes further, from the bladder, via the ureter, to the kidney, causing kidney infections. In women the bladder infection cystitis is the most common UTI, while in men it is urethritis (inflammation of the urethra). Symptoms may be absent or include frequent urination, painful urination or abdominal pain. Antibiotic treatment is usually successful, although bacteria such as *E. coli* can form biofilms in the bladder that are particularly resistant to the action of the immune system and antibiotics, and cause recurrent infections.

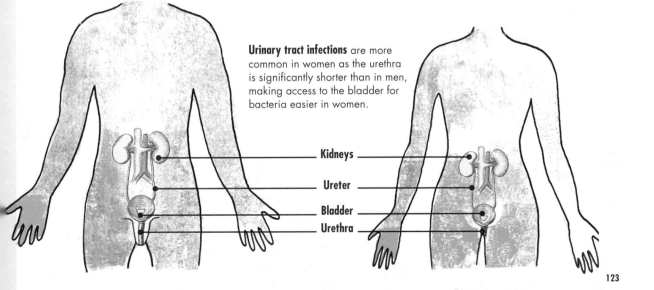

Urinary tract infections are more common in women as the urethra is significantly shorter than in men, making access to the bladder for bacteria easier in women.

Kidneys

Ureter

Bladder

Urethra

WHAT THE GOOD BACTERIA DO FOR US

The star of the show in the vagina is *Lactobacillus*, the dominant bacterial species by a long way. Several *Lactobacillus* species lower the pH of the vagina to 3.5–4 by producing copious amounts of lactic acid, a major factor in controlling the growth of bacteria that cause bacterial vaginosis, sexually transmitted diseases, urinary infections and premature birth.

There are hints emerging that women who have a low proportion of *Lactobacillus* bacteria in their fallopian tubes and/or uterus may be more prone to ectopic pregnancies and miscarriage. In a study of women who had in vitro fertilization, a shift from a *Lactobacillus*-dominant to a non-*Lactobacillus*-dominant community of bacteria in the uterus corresponded to diminished implantation rates and increased miscarriage risk.

The role of Lactobacillus bacteria in the vagina
(1) *Lactobacillus* produce lactic acid to maintain pH at less than 4.5. (2) Thanks to their high numbers, they outcompete pathogenic bacteria. (3) *Lactobacillus* down-regulate inflammatory cytokines. (4) They also kill bacteria by producing hydrogen peroxide, (5) and other molecules. (6) *Lactobacillus* break down bacterial biofilms.

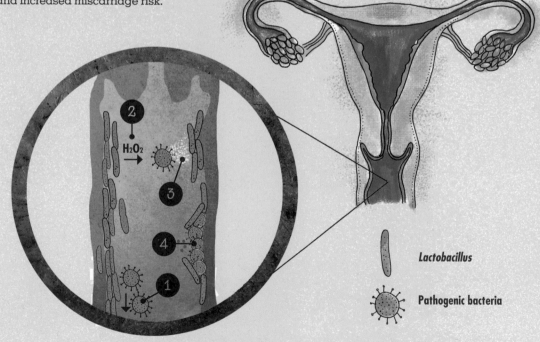

H_2O_2

Lactobacillus

Pathogenic bacteria

In men, the two main controllable factors that impact on the bacterial health of the penis are sexual practices and circumcision.

MAKING THE CUT

Circumcision — the surgical removal of the foreskin — is routinely carried out in some countries for religious reasons and sometimes for medical ones. Worldwide about 40 percent of men are circumcised, with around 10 percent in European and nearer 100 percent in Muslim and Jewish populations.

Circumcision can be a disturbing procedure for the bacterial world. In sharp contrast to other areas of the body, the reduction in both total number and the diversity of bacteria is beneficial here. Circumcision reduces the risk of contracting the HIV virus by at least 50 percent, probably because it preferentially removes the anaerobic bacteria (for example, *Prevotella*, *Dialister*, *Finegoldia* and *Peptoniphilus*)

that are associated with an increased HIV risk. These bacteria living under the foreskin can cause minor inflammatory immune responses that stimulate the immune cells (CD4+ T cells) infected with HIV, allowing AIDS to develop.

In circumcised men these anaerobic bacteria are significantly reduced in number and diversity. Practising safe sex remains the best HIV-prevention strategy, but topical creams that adjust the balance of bacteria on the penis might some day help to lower the risk of infection.

LACTOBACILLUS
FULLY DOCUMENTED 1900
CRISPATUS

GRAM-POSITIVE ROD

WHAT:
One of the *Lactobacillus* bacterial family, most commonly associated with the fermentation of milk to make cheese and yogurt and vegetables to make sauerkraut.

WHERE:
Normal inhabitant of the vagina.

HOW:
L. crispatus produces lactic acid, a potent broad spectrum antibacterial and antiviral agent.

CASE NOTES:
Up to 30 percent of new HIV cases in women might be averted if *Lactobacillus* species such as *L. crispatus* dominated in the vaginal bacterial community. The bacterium is also implicated in the control of bacterial vaginosis.

ENCOURAGING THE GOOD AND DISCOURAGING THE BAD

Daily habits (sexual, dietary and personal hygiene) all play a part in STD and UTI risk. Although one in five women will develop a UTI at some point in their lives, most men will never have a UTI, with an incidence of well below 1 percent. However, in sexually active people bacteria are routinely shared, so the pressure is on to keep bacteria such as *E.coli* and *C. trachomatis* under control.

CONDOMS

Tests for STDs are recommended for anyone who has regular unprotected sex (that is, sex without a condom), particularly if they have multiple partners or when they meet a new partner. Condoms are widely available and often free; their use can prevent STDs, and in some cases UTIs in both men and women.

Anyone unlucky enough to have had a UTI will remember that burning sensation and unremitting need to pee. But there are ways to help avoid a second dose.

TOILET HABITS

Concentrated urine encourages UTI so drinking lots of water helps, as does the regular passing of a dilute urine — the most likely way to flush out any pathogenic bacteria. So urination after sex is also recommended. And if you need to go, go! Holding it in just gives those bad bacteria time to grow.

Bowel habits are pretty important too. Constipation makes it difficult to empty your bladder totally, meaning trapped bacteria have plenty of time to grow and cause infection. On the other hand, diarrhea is also not a good thing, as loose stools increase the chances of a pathogenic bacterium making its way into the vagina or urethra. Wiping is key here — front to back is the way to do it.

A UROGENITAL-FRIENDLY DIET

Having healthy gut bacteria has knock-on effects for the whole body, as well as for UTIs and STDs, so eat well, with plenty of fiber in the form of fruit and vegetables. Some of these seem to be particularly beneficial for genital health. In women who are prone to vaginosis, eating citrus fruits, tomatoes and strawberries, with high levels of Vitamin C, may help to prevent a recurrence. Using apple cider vinegar on a salad is also a good way to prevent UTIs, as the acetic acid it contains inhibits the growth of *E. coli*.

Home remedies for UTIs, STDs and vaginosis range from consuming yogurt and garlic — a well-known antibacterial — to drinking cranberry juice. While many women swear by cranberry juice for UTIs, the science is a little murky. Studies have shown that it does not contain enough of the active ingredient to be very effective. It is also loaded with sugar, so probably not a great addition to your diet.

DIETARY SUPPLEMENTS

D-mannose powder, a sugar extracted from fruit, is attracting attention as a more natural way than antibiotics to manage UTIs. D-mannose is not absorbed very well by the body, but passes through the kidneys and ends up in the bladder, where it can help get rid of *E.coli* (see graphic).

A few studies have demonstrated a potential use for probiotics (see pages 160–61) to prevent female UTI and vaginal disease, but success has been limited. This is possibly because the community of bacteria varies from woman to woman. Future approaches could therefore include personalized probiotics. Strains of bacteria such as the beneficial *Lactobacillus rhamnosus* GR-1 can survive the passage through the digestive tract and go on to colonize the vagina and bladder.

Yogurt is rich in probiotics, especially plain Greek yogurt. Yeast infections such as thrush can be controlled by eating such *Lactobacillus*-containing yogurt regularly. Some health practitioners even advocate inserting a small amount of yogurt into the vagina, but it's probably worth checking with your doctor on that one!

KEEPING YOUR COOL

Cotton or natural fibers are best for underwear: synthetic fabrics do not allow the skin to breathe, and the resulting excessive moisture encourages bacteria to grow. If you're tempted by thongs, remember that thin and chafing G-strings are likely to result in more discomfort, as they easily transfer bacteria from rectum to vagina.

Changing sanitary protection regularly is a must: soiled sanitary pads and tampons are places where bacteria can grow very easily. In the worst-case scenario toxic shock syndrome occurs when there is an overgrowth of *Staphylococcus aureus*, usually when a tampon has been left in place longer than the recommended time of 8 hours.

Good hygiene is important, but douching is not recommended. Flushing water or douches into the vagina upsets the pH balance, making it too alkaline and killing off beneficial bacteria. However, in uncircumcised men, cleaning gently under the foreskin with mild soap and water is also a good way of minimizing the build-up of potential pathogens.

How does D-mannose work in your bladder to treat UTI?

(1) Sugar molecules on the bladder cell wall.

(2) *E. coli* (the principal cause of UTI) clings to the sugar molecules.

(3) After taking D-mannose supplements (orange), *E. coli* preferentially attaches to it and is flushed out of the bladder in the urine.

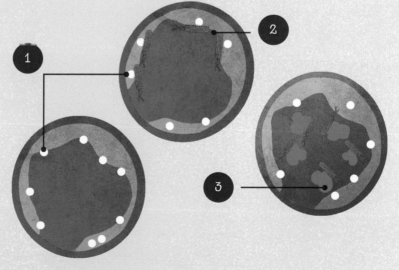

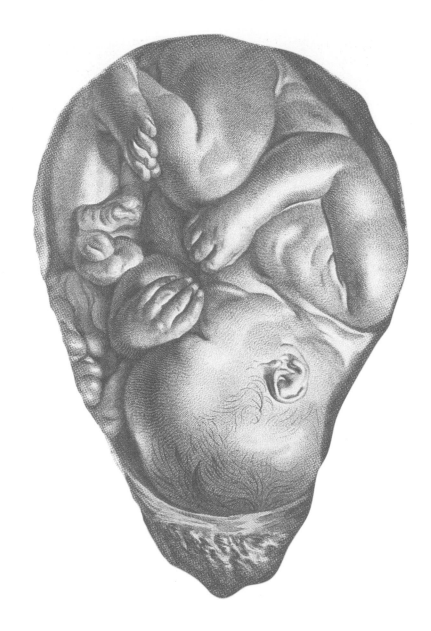

PREGNANCY AND BEYOND

In the first few hours of life, a baby transforms from being mostly human to being mostly bacterial — in terms of cell number, that is. The first few bacteria the baby swallows in the womb, as it emerges into the world and during the first year or so of life, are providing food for thought, both for mothers and health professionals. Encouraging friendly bacteria from the start is now thought to have significant long-term health benefits.

PREGNANCY FROM A MOTHER'S PERSPECTIVE

Pregnant women are bombarded by health advice on the right diet, the use of medicines and the management of chronic health conditions, not to mention the increased risk of certain infections. Sexually transmitted diseases and bacterial urinary tract infections can be harmful to both mother and baby. Many other infections of concern in pregnancy are caused by a virus or the toxoplasma parasite, but others, such as listeria food poisoning and streptococcal sepsis, are on the bacterial list.

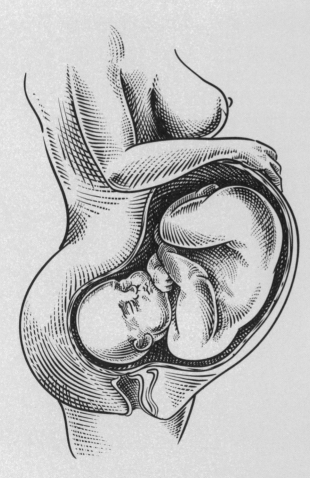

Pregnant women are almost 20 times more likely to develop listeriosis than the rest of the population because the body's immune response to the *Listeria monocytogenes* bacteria weakens during pregnancy. This is an interesting downside of pregnancy as a whole. The baby is an alien from an immunologic point of view — or at least the half driven by its father's genes is — so many immune responses are naturally dampened down to prevent the baby being rejected (in the way that transplanted organs may be rejected). Listeria in pregnancy does not usually pose a serious threat to the mother's health. However, it can cause complications around pregnancy and birth or result in miscarriage. Avoiding soft cheeses and pâté is thus recommended.

Encased in the womb, the baby is protected, although even here bacteria exert subtle effects on the developing baby and on the mother too.

Lysteria monocytogenes

Group B *Streptococcus* bacteria are carried by up to 30 percent of people, but rarely cause symptoms. In a small number of pregnancies, they infect the baby just before or during labor, leading to sepsis and sometimes stillbirth. Although this is still relatively uncommon, cases are on the rise and it has been suggested that women should be routinely tested. The burden of this infection worldwide, particularly in developing countries, is such that the emphasis is now shifting from prophylactic antibiotic use to the development of vaccines for maternal immunization.

A SHIFTING LANDSCAPE

Avoiding pathogenic bacteria is important for a healthy pregnancy. However, behind the scenes, the commensal bacteria in a pregnant mother's body undergo subtle changes. The bacteria found in the vaginas of pregnant women are different from those in non-pregnant women. Although high numbers of *Lactobacilli* are still present, there is a shift toward species normally only found in the gut, to provide the baby with the best possible start in life. As the baby is born these become some of the early gut colonizers, getting the baby ready for the diet of the next few months and beyond.

The gut microbiome also shifts in pregnant women toward a less diverse state. It seems this may be one of the reasons behind the weight gain seen in pregnancy. Germ-free mice given a transplant of human third-trimester bacteria gained more weight and had higher levels of glucose in the blood. As in some obese individuals, the metabolism in pregnancy ratchets up a level to glean every ounce of nutrition from food, and such bacterial changes may contribute to this.

After the baby is born, its mother's microbiome slowly returns to normal. Shifting the baby weight is always tricky, but breastfeeding seems to help, partly by burning up additional stored calories. It is not yet known whether breastfeeding also reverses the obesity-like bacterial changes of pregnancy, but it does reduce the risk of Type 2 diabetes and heart disease later in life. All of this is likely to be mediated by a change in the gut bacteria.

Even in the shifting landscapes of pregnancy, the helpful and protective *Lactobacillus* bacteria (pink in this image) dominate in the vagina.

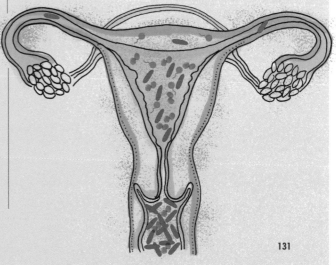

131

A BABY'S PERSPECTIVE

The nine months that it takes a human baby to develop and grow in the womb is a long time potentially to influence its development and future health. The womb was once thought to be a sterile environment, but we now know that there are bacteria associated with the placenta and in the amniotic fluid.

However, this finding is so new that it is not entirely clear what role these bacteria play. Certainly the bacteria are swallowed by the baby, and these early colonizers of its gut are the same bacteria that show up in meconium — the baby's first bowel movement.

The initial exposure of the fetus in the womb to bacteria primes the immune system and the gut epithelium to respond appropriately to pathogenic and commensal bacterial after birth. Exposure to

these bacteria during pregnancy may be an even more important influence on the development of allergies (and possible other diseases) than the gut profile during the early months of life.

One area attracting a lot of interest is epigenetics. This concerns how DNA, our genetic material, can be modified by environmental factors to turn genes on or off, such as the deprivation of key nutrients in famine situations. It is a complex area, but one

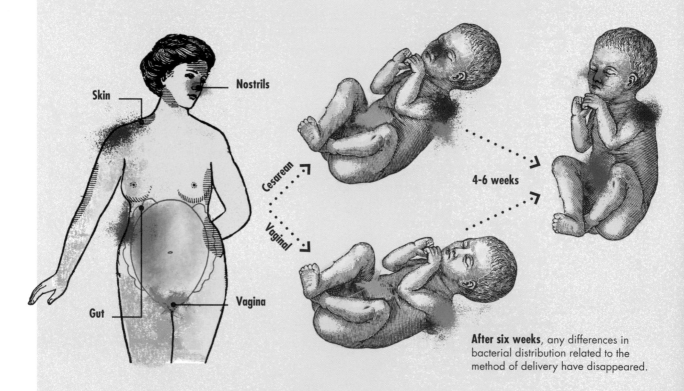

After six weeks, any differences in bacterial distribution related to the method of delivery have disappeared.

that is relevant here because some human studies have shown that exposure to certain bacteria in the womb can result in epigenetic modifications to our immune system. And these modifications can be inheritable — an unconventional finding as it challenges the idea that inheritance only occurs through the DNA code that passes from parent to offspring. Many studies are investigating the effects of diet and bacterial infections on the gut microbiome and the ways in which these translate to epigenetic changes, influencing anything from the development of the fetal brain to its predisposition to cancer as an adult.

The early composition of a baby's gut bacteria can be affected by a mother's diet or health status. Interestingly, in babies born to diabetic mothers, the meconium bacterial diversity varies according to how well controlled the mother's blood sugar levels were — just one example of how a mother's diet in pregnancy may affect a newborn's gut bacteria.

HOW WE ACQUIRE OUR MICROBIOME

Cesarean births are increasingly common. In the U.K. some 25 percent of births are by cesarean and in the U.S. it is closer to 33 percent, with rates near 50 percent in countries such as China, Brazil and Turkey. There are concerns about this level of surgical intervention, but also a recognition that it is related to the general fall in infant and maternal mortality worldwide.

Within minutes of being born vaginally, a baby starts to acquire more bacteria. Many different species of bacteria can be detected all over a baby when it is born, with no site-specific pattern, unlike in adults. Not surprisingly, the most important early colonizers are the predominant members of the vaginal and skin bacteria of the mother, namely *Lactobacillus*, *Propionibacterium*, *Streptococcus* and *Staphylococcus*. These are present across all the body sites in a newborn baby. In contrast, the baby's meconium only contains species that are gut-specific such as *Escherichia* and *Klebsiella*. These are not seen in any other body site in a newborn and are probably acquired in the womb.

So does it matter, in terms of your early bacterial guests, if you are born by cesarean rather than vaginal delivery? Probably not — or at least not for long. In a recent study minor variations in the bacteria of newborns delivered by cesarean were found in some sites, such as the mouth and skin. But the latest research suggests that any effects of delivery method are short-lived. By six weeks of age these differences disappear and the bacterial profile is primarily driven by the environmental conditions of a specific site rather than by mode of delivery. What happens next, in terms of the baby's diet, may be more relevant. A number of factors have been studied that may influence the very early microbiome of the infant gut: gestational age (whether a baby is full term or premature), maternal and infant obesity, maternal diet (fat intake), maternal gestational diabetes and breastfeeding. We do not know precisely how influential some of these are, but how a baby is fed in its early weeks and months is significant.

In an added twist, the onset of labor prior to delivery, rather than the cesarean procedure itself, may have the greatest impact on the maternal origin of the bacteria on newborns. Babies born by emergency cesarean performed after women had already been in labor had a bacterial profile derived from maternal vaginal and skin bacteria (similar to vaginally delivered babies), whereas the bacteria of planned cesarean babies' was mainly skin-derived. The need for an emergency delivery may be related to an underlying maternal or fetal medical condition — one that could, in itself, affect maternal and/or fetal bacteria.

FOOD FOR BACTERIA

In the first few weeks of life, the bacterial community all over the body diversifies and becomes site specific, but the gut has a particular focus early on. The gut bacteria of a newborn baby are most closely related to those of the mother's vagina, although the bacteria are much less diverse in the vagina than in the mother's gut.

A vagina that has such a limited diversity seems curious, when diversity is the name of the game elsewhere in the body. But the *Lactobacillus* species in the vagina are very good news for the baby for three reasons.

Breast is best because it not only contains all the right nutrients for a developing baby but also for the bacteria in its gut.

Firstly, these *Lactobacillus* crowd out any unfriendly bacteria as the baby's gut begins to be colonized. Secondly, they kill off any nasty bacteria. And finally, and most importantly considering the limited nature of a newborn's diet, they digest the lactose found in milk.

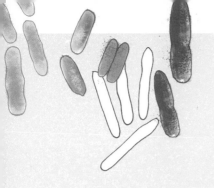

BREAST IS BEST

A balanced bacterial community, particularly in the gut, can guard against all sorts of diseases. Children who develop the autoimmune disease Type 1 diabetes, for example, have abnormalities in their gut microbiomes. A healthy gut microbiome can help to protect against asthma and IBD throughout life. We know from animal models of disease that if you get the good bacteria into your gut early on, you increase your chances of being healthy later in life.

A recent study showed that 30 percent of the beneficial bacteria in a baby's gut come directly from mother's milk and an additional 10 percent from skin on the mother's breast. The origin of breast milk bacteria remains unclear, but they may travel to the breast from the mother's gut. Amazingly, there are at least 700 bacterial species present in breast milk.

As if providing the nutrients, lactose and fat, as well as helping to seed the baby's gut were not enough, human breast milk uniquely contains more than two hundred human milk oligosaccharides (HMOs). Remarkably, adult humans cannot digest these, but a bacterium in the baby's gut can. *Bifidobacterium longum infantis* outcompetes any other bacteria in the gut, providing that it gets its tasty HMOs. In return it performs many helpful tasks, training and regulating the immune response; it may even be involved in the rapid growth of the human brain during the first year of life.

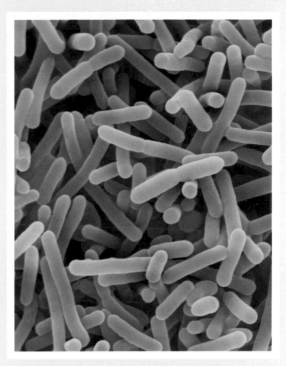

***Bifidobacterium* bacteria:** one species of these, B. infantis, is unique among gut bacteria in its ability to digest human milk oligosaccharides (a class of carbohydrates).

WHAT HAPPENS DURING WEANING

For the first three years of a child's life, the gut bacteria are pretty unstable, so there is plenty of scope to influence what is there. The greatest changes take place at 9–18 months, when solid foods are increasingly introduced. In one experiment, introducing lots of vegetables such as peas and broccoli produced a switch from a gut dominated by *Acitinobacteria* and *Proteobacteria* to one dominated by *Firmicutes* and *Bacterioides*. By three years old, the high levels of *Lactobacilli* in the child's gut and any early differences brought about by breast or formula feeding have waned.

THE BEST START IN LIFE

The method of delivery does not seem to have a long-term effect on the development of a baby's microbiome. However, there are ways to modulate your child's microbiome that might give him or her the best start in life.

EARLY NUTRITION

Breast milk is the best, most natural foodstuff for the first six months of life and then for up to a year alongside solid food. Yet, according to a recent study the U.K. has the lowest rate of breastfeeding in the world, especially in later months, while in the U.S. the number of breastfeeding newborns has risen recently, although many mothers stop after six months. The pressure is on, both to support women and to increase breastfeeding rates, as well as to advise on the best formula milk for mothers unable to breastfeed.

GOODNESS IN EVERY DROP

Breast milk changes in composition to meet the baby's needs and contains many nutritional and immunological components.

- WATER
- PROTEINS
- LACTOSE
- FATTY ACIDS
- VITAMINS & MINERALS
- HORMONES & GROWTH FACTORS

- STEM CELLS
- AT LEAST 700 STRAINS OF BACTERIA
- IMMUNE SYSTEM CELLS, ANTIBODIES
- ANTIBACTERIAL & ANTIVIRAL ENZYMES

Infant formulas, usually based on cow's milk, are highly regulated and designed to mimic the nutritional composition of breast milk as closely as possible. Many formula milks, reflecting the changing approach to bacteria, now contain prebiotics, and some contain probiotics too. More research is needed to determine the long-term effects of feeding infants probiotic-laced formula, but these probiotics may be a welcome addition.

Reassuringly, although the benefits of breastfeeding are cumulative, the gain is significant even if you can only breastfeed for the first few days. The first milk produced by the mother, colostrum, is rich in antibodies that will protect against bacterial diseases. Transfer of protective bacteria happens the moment that the baby starts feeding.

A BABY-FRIENDLY DIET

Encouraging a healthy gut microbiome is a prime focus, for both mother and baby, and diet is a big factor. There are no surprises here: providing plenty of fruit and vegetables to nourish those fiber-loving bacteria is beneficial both for pregnant mothers' gut bacteria and for babies when they are weaned. The Mediterranean diet wins every time (see page 113).

Breast milk is sweet due to its lactose content, which is why babies naturally like sweet things. However, the more you can persuade them that a spoonful of broccoli is delicious, the more you can encourage good gut bacteria. Early and constant exposure to a wide range of colorful fruit and vegetables — starting with fruits, then moving via sweet vegetables such as carrots and parsnips to the more bitter broccoli and spinach — encourages a diet for a happy and healthy (bacterial) life. Smuggled inside tomato sauces, finely chopped if necessary and widely eaten by the rest of the family, a Mediterranean, vegetable-based diet can only be a good thing.

BACTERIAL KILLERS

Women are routinely given antibiotic treatments in pregnancy and labor and often for very good reasons — for example, in cases of a previous history of Group B *Streptococcus* infection — but antibiotics should only be used by mothers and babies when strictly necessary. They are not bad in themselves, but the perils of antibiotic resistance and the disruption to beneficial bacteria are well documented.

Probiotics in general and taken after antibiotic treatment may be the way forward. They boost the good bacteria and are generally considered safe in pregnancy, whether taken vaginally or orally, and when breastfeeding. Probiotics include bacteria such as *Lactobacillus rhamnosus* strain GG, *Lactobacillus reuteri* and *Bifidobacterium lacti*. One strain of *Lactobacillus paracasei* has also been attracting attention, after studies in mice showed that administration of this probiotic to pregnant or lactating mice could prevent allergies developing in their offspring.

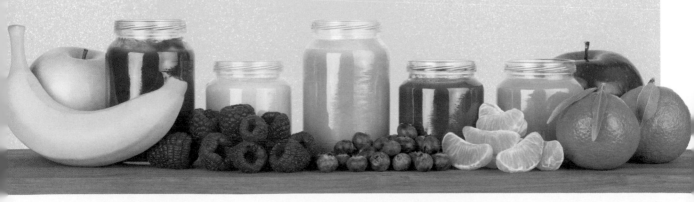

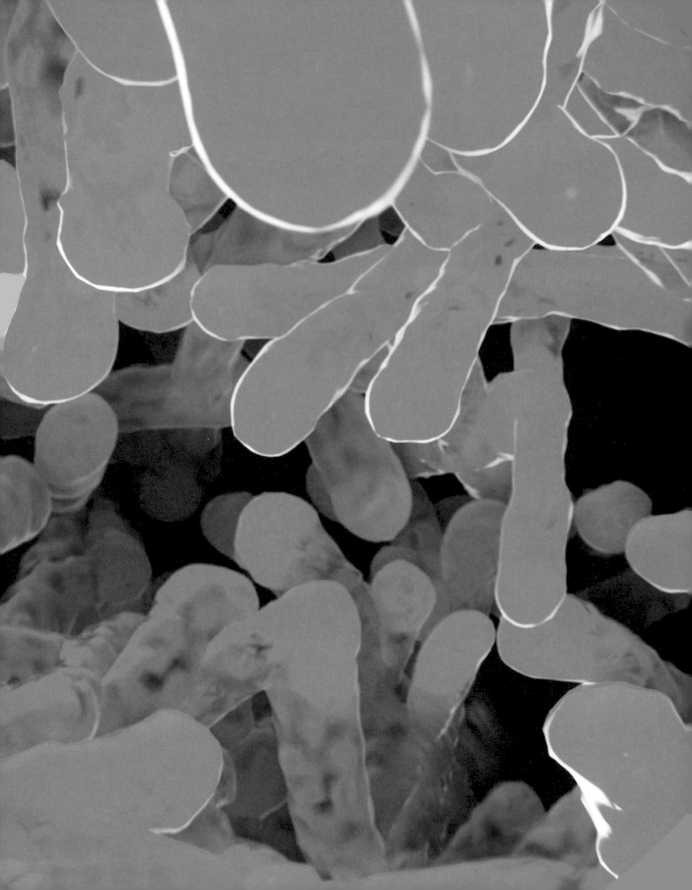

CHAPTER THREE

TO BOLDLY GO

You have been introduced to your bacteria, what they do and how they have become the most successful group of organisms on the planet — as well as which parts of your body they like to inhabit. This chapter explores how your actions influence these communities of bacteria and how they, in turn, affect you. We look at how you can change your bacteria — your commensal guests as well as those that live in your home and at your office — for better health. Perhaps most importantly, each topic in this chapter features new and different thinking about bacteria. No longer viewed as germs to be killed, many are now understood to be valued guests of honor that require attention and nurturing. Your health depends on it.

Bacillus **(capital "B")** refers to a specific group of bacteria, whereas bacillus refers to the rod-like shape of bacteria. The bacteria in this image are bacillus, but not necessarily *Bacillus*.

DISCOVERING NEW BACTERIA

Although the discovery of new species of bacteria is relatively rare, microbiologists have estimated that there are at least ten thousand, and there may be more than one million species of bacteria on Earth. It is a large range, due in part to controversy over what constitutes a "species."

A species is defined as a group of organisms capable of having offspring that can also have offspring, usually through sexual reproduction. Bacteria break a few of these rules by dividing mainly by asexual reproduction (fission, see page 28) and by their ability to incorporate foreign DNA (from another species or even as diverse a group as a virus or fungus) into their own genome (see page 29).

Despite looking very different, all domestic dogs belong to the same species (*Canis lupus familiaris*), whereas the two different species of bacteria shown here — *Lactobacillus acidophilus* and *Lactobacillus delbrueckii* — look identical.

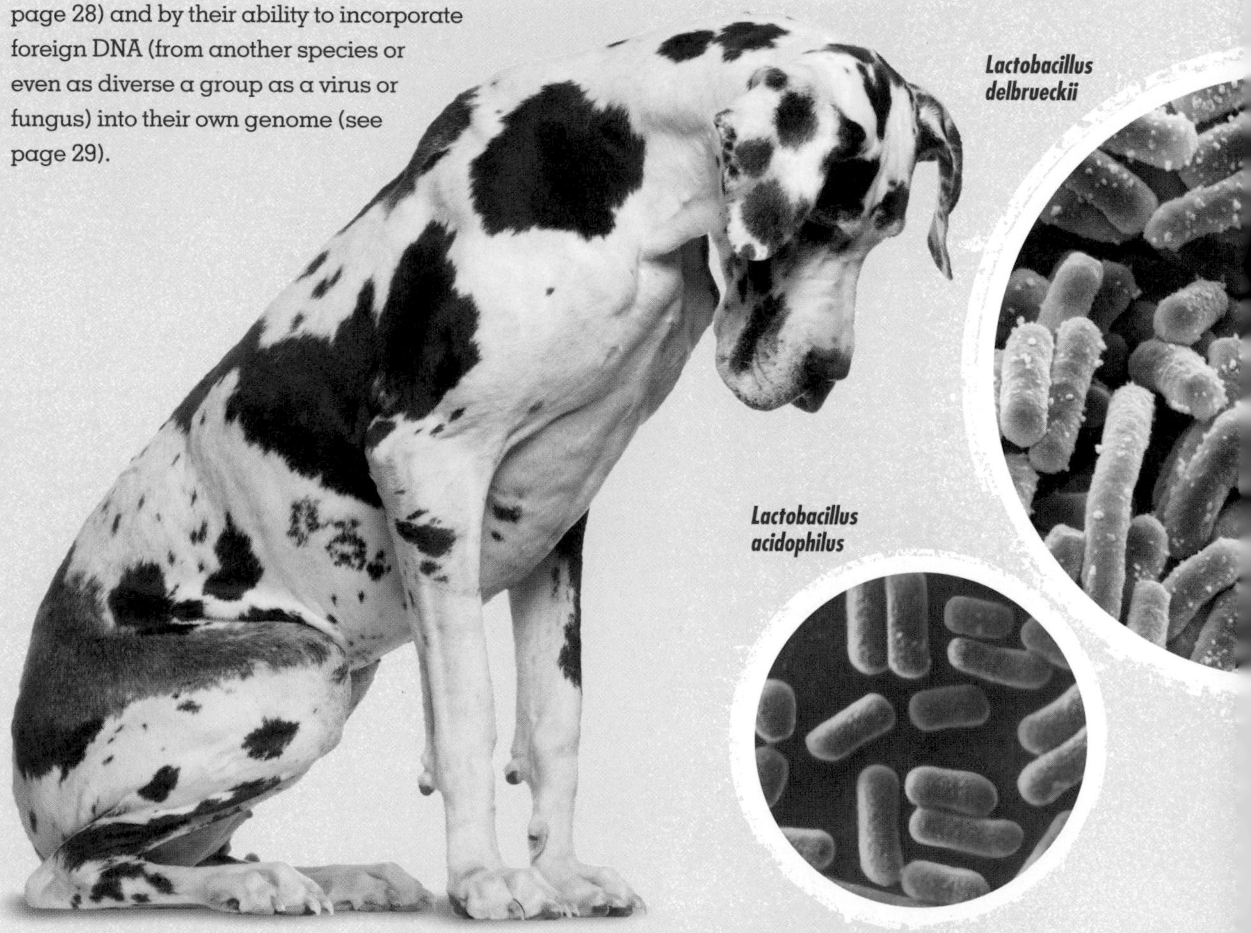

Lactobacillus delbrueckii

Lactobacillus acidophilus

Scientists searching for new bacteria sample a habitat (sea water, for example), remove all DNA in the sample and then use a specific region of that DNA for identification — much like a barcode. They can compare the "barcodes" with a database to understand which known species are present and which are new to science. This system is very useful for indicating diversity, but does not tell scientists much about the organisms themselves. Imagine shopping in a supermarket using only barcodes — you can see that there are many different products, but know little else about them.

The bacteria that make newspaper headlines are generally new strains rather than new species (see page 17). For example, a patient may have a new, more virulent strain of some type of bacterial infection. Some are more headline-grabbing than others, such as *Halomonas titanicae*, found to be munching its way through the rusting hulk of that iconic ship at the bottom of the North Atlantic.

DISCOVERING NEW SPECIES

The last decade has seen the discovery of some exciting new species of bacteria:

Plastic bottle eaters: Japanese scientists took samples from different areas of a plastic bottle recycling site and discovered *Ideonella sakaiensis*, which was producing an enzyme that broke down the plastic for "food."

Oil-lovers: About 30 different types of bacteria, some of which might be entirely new species, have been found living in shale oil and gas wells used for hydraulic fracturing or "fracking." One species, named *Candidatus frackibacter*, is thought to be unique to these sites.

Disease causers: A new species, *Borrelia mayonii*, was discovered to be the culprit in new cases of Lyme disease in the U.S. in 2016. Originally Lyme disease was thought to be caused solely by the species *Borrelia burgdorferi*, but scientists studying the genome of *B. burgdorferi* at the Mayo Clinic in Minnesota discovered that some genes in their sample were quite different. They declared a new species, which they duly named after the Mayo Clinic — *B. mayonii*.

Nano-sized bacteria: Scientists in Colorado who strained groundwater through an incredibly fine filter discovered 35 new groups of bacteria. These were smaller than any bacteria known to science, some being only 400 nanometers (less than half a micron) across. The new groups are still being described and may represent a new branch on the evolutionary tree (see pages 12–13).

NEW THINKING ABOUT BACTERIA

Not surprisingly, as more has been discovered about bacteria, our thinking about them has also changed. The scientific community has spent decades identifying the "bad bacteria" responsible for human diseases; the medical mantra was "find the bug, find the drug." However, such thinking is limited and fails to consider the healthy community of bacteria upon which we humans (and potentially all life) depend. A new approach was required.

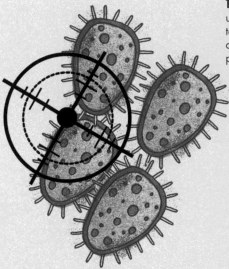

Traditional thinking was to target bad bugs, usually at the expense of good bacteria. Modern techniques have shifted to promoting healthy and diverse communities of good bacteria, which can prevent bad bugs from colonizing.

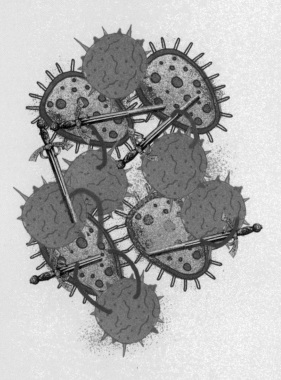

Looking at communities of bacteria, both good and bad, rather than just "bad bugs" requires a much broader perspective on health. Cleaning up a "bad neighborhood" does not simply mean arresting the bad guys, but involves exploring the neighborhood as a whole to understand what has enabled them to thrive there. This fundamental shift to thinking about bacteria as an entire community has influenced scientific approaches over the last few decades.

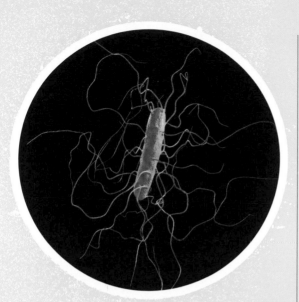

Clostridium difficile

THE CASE OF
CLOSTRIDIUM DIFFICILE

The change in how persistent *Clostridium difficile* infections are treated is a great example of how our thinking about bacteria has progressed. People often acquire a *C. difficile* infection during or after treatment with a general antibiotic for another type of infection. The symptoms are diarrhea, painful stomach cramps, nausea, loss of appetite and dehydration — not ideal when you are recovering from another infection. In the past those infected with *C. difficile* would be given another antibiotic (sometimes before they had finished the first course of antibiotics for the original infection). The second course was generally sufficient to clear up the *C. difficile* infection in about three-quarters of patients, but the remaining one-quarter then suffered a second infection of *C. difficile* after antibiotic treatment ended.

Traditionally more antibiotics would have been used to target this persistent bug. However, new thinking suggests that it is an imbalance in the bacterial community that allows *C. difficile* to continue to thrive. The gut microbiomes of patients with recurrent *C. difficile* infections show a much lower diversity of bacteria than completely healthy people or those whose *C. difficile* infection cleared up with the first antibiotic treatment. Therefore, instead of giving patients with recurring infections repeated courses of antibiotics, physicians are now prescribing a healthy and diverse community of bacteria — in the form of a fecal transplant (see page 163).

THINKING OUTSIDE THE PETRI DISH

While the idea that bacteria in your stomach can affect your mood (see pages 150–51) or train your immune system (see pages 38–39) might seem rather weird to most of us, some "outside the box" theories under discussion among the scientific community are pushing the scientific envelope still further.

Petri dishes are used to culture bacteria in the laboratory. The bottom of the shallow dish is filled with a jelly-like substance (agar) that is infused with nutrients to feed the bacteria, while the lid prevents contamination.

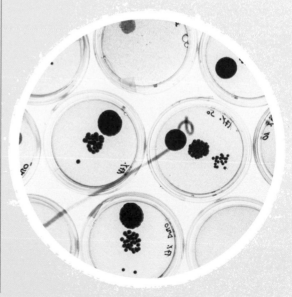

BACTERIA AND CANCER

While some bad bacteria have been linked with an increased risk of cancer — *Chlamydia trachomatis* and cervical cancer, for example — scientists are now exploring ways of recruiting bacteria to help fight other forms of cancer. Researchers at the Massachusetts Institute of Technology (MIT) and the University of California in San Diego, programmed *E. coli* to deliver cancer-treating drugs to tumor sites. The scientists took advantage of the fact that bacteria naturally gather at tumor sites to deliver specific chemicals directly to the cancerous cells. Tests so far have been on mice only, but it is an interesting new approach to cancer treatment.

BACTERIA WITH BRAINS

Scientists in the U.S. have proposed that bacteria are smarter than we might think, based on how they respond to their environment. Bacteria have different types of receptors on their cell surfaces that bind with different molecules in their environment. The greater the variety of receptors that a bacterium possesses, the more it is able to understand its environment and respond accordingly. The most commonly studied bacterium, *E. coli*, is apparently relatively unintelligent with only five types of receptors. In contrast the soil bacterium *Azospirillum brasilense* has 48 different types of receptors, making it a bacterial "genius."

VIRUS PUPPET MASTERS

There is another character that might have a bigger say in the health of your microbiome than your human cells — the bacteriophage. This is a virus that specializes in attacking bacteria. Three-quarters of people around the world play host to a bacteriophage known as crAssphage, which infects the most common group of bacteria in the human gut, the *Bacteroides*. This bacteriophage is more ubiquitous among humans than any single species of bacteria. The research on crAssphage is still in its early stages, but researchers have hypothesized that it may be responsible for controlling the diversity of bacteria in your gut, playing puppet master to the bacteria of your microbiome. Makes you wonder who is in control of whom?

In 2017, scientists discovered that there is a whole crAss-like family of phages associated with the human microbiome.

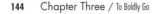

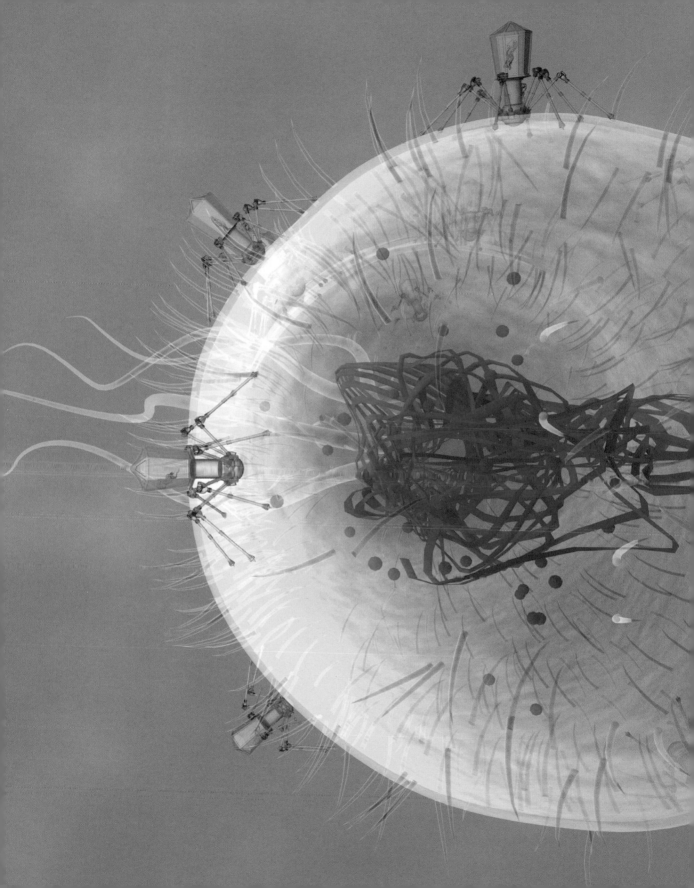

DIET AND GUT BACTERIA

What you eat directly affects the health of your gut bacteria, making diet the single biggest influence on gut health. Just as the type of soil or amount of rain and sun determines what plants can grow in a habitat, so the food you eat determines which species of bacteria will flourish in your gut.

Just like your human cells, bacterial cells need a healthy, balanced diet. The best fuel for your gut bacteria is fiber, the indigestible part of plant-based foods. Your gut bacteria ferment this fiber into molecules that you can digest, essentially extracting calories from it that you are unable to extract on your own.

A diet high in fiber is the best way to keep your gut bacteria happy; when the bacteria do not get enough fiber, the bacteria starve and die off.

CHANGING DIET

It does not take long for your gut bacteria to change in response to what you eat. You can increase the relative amounts of fiber-fermenting bacteria, for example, within 24 hours of increasing the fiber content of your diet. Over a matter of weeks, these changes can start to affect your health. A study in 2015 swapped the diets of African-Americans (generally a high-fat, low-fiber Western diet) and rural Africans (a low-fat, high-fiber diet); it took only two weeks for the gut bacteria in both groups to change. The African-Americans had more fiber-fermenting bacteria, an increase in the short-chain fatty acids that protect against cancer, and less inflammation of the gut lining. The rural Africans on the Western diet experienced the opposite.

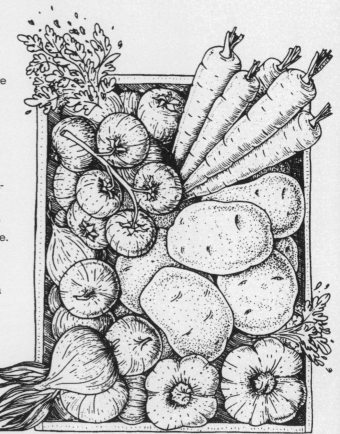

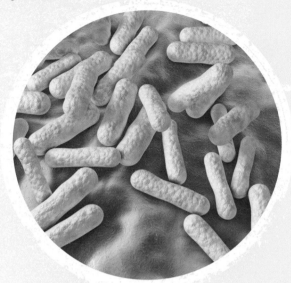

Zobellia galactanivorans

YOUR BACTERIA ARE WHAT YOU EAT

The marine bacteria *Zobellia galactanivorans* feed on red algae, producing a special enzyme that breaks down the algae's tough cell walls. When people in Japan ate the red algae, they naturally also consumed some of the *Zobellia* found on it. These marine bacteria would not have found a human gut a favorable place to live and probably did not survive for long. However, at some stage bacteria that *do* enjoy the habitat of the human gut, *Bacteroides plebeius*, must have managed to incorporate the gene that produces the enzyme that destroys cell walls into their genome. So although *Bacteroides plebeius* is found in human guts around the world, the only strain capable of breaking down seaweed is found in Japanese people.

THE ATHLETIC GUT

Research has been undertaken to establish links between the microbiome and athletic ability and is uncovering a link between activity and microbial make-up. Scientists at the APC Microbiome Institute in Cork, Ireland, published papers reporting their findings that the gut flora of professional Irish rugby players was more diverse than that of a healthy control group. Research is ongoing into how gut bacteria in elite athletes helps them to process food better, reduce inflammation and perform with greater efficiency. It takes guts to be a top athlete, it seems.

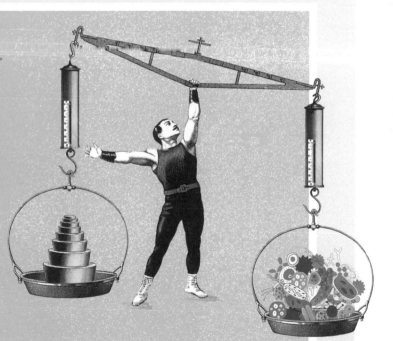

GUT BACTERIA AND YOUR HEALTH

The profound effect of diet upon your gut bacteria is not yet fully understood. Scientists are still unsure whether food itself is directly responsible for changing the bacterial community or whether something more complicated is happening. They are also trying to unravel how these different communities in the gut might affect human health. While many links have been found between unhappy gut bacteria and disease, it remains unclear in which direction these links flow. Does disease change your gut bacteria, or do changes in gut bacteria cause disease?

While there may be no such thing as the "ideal" gut community, scientists agree that diversity is a sign of a healthy and happy gut: the more species of bacteria the better. Eating a variety of high-fiber foods, rich in antioxidants, such as blueberries, raspberries, artichokes and kidney beans, promotes a diverse gut community.

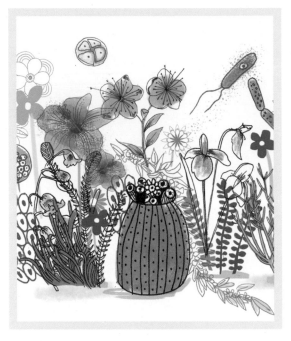

A happy, healthy gut has a rich diversity of bacteria

TREATMENT

Encouraging the growth of good bacteria using prebiotics and probiotics (see pages 160–61), and transferring good bacteria from healthy people to patients through fecal transplants (see page 163) are both being explored as treatments for disease. Although the connections between gut bacteria and different diseases are still being made, the hope is that this research will lead to new treatments (see page 107).

LOSING DIVERSITY

When a student examined how his gut microbes had changed after a strict diet of fast food for two weeks, he found that he had lost around 40 percent (1,400 species) of the species diversity.

WITHOUT YOUR GUT BACTERIA, SCIENTISTS ESTIMATE THAT YOU WOULD GET 10–15 PERCENT FEWER CALORIES FROM THE SAME AMOUNT OF FOOD

Antioxidants found in tea slow the growth of bad bacteria in the gut, but do not affect your good gut microbes.

BACTERIA AND MOOD

In the 19th century it was thought that the wastes that build up in your colon could produce toxins; these in turn made you depressed, anxious and even psychotic. While anxiety is (thankfully) no longer treated with colonic purges, scientists are accumulating evidence that the bacteria living in your intestines can influence your mood and, ultimately, your mental health.

People with serious depression tend to have fewer and less diverse species of bacteria in their gut microbiome than those free from it. But we do not yet know whether this change in the microbiome is a cause of depression or a consequence of it — the chicken and egg conundrum.

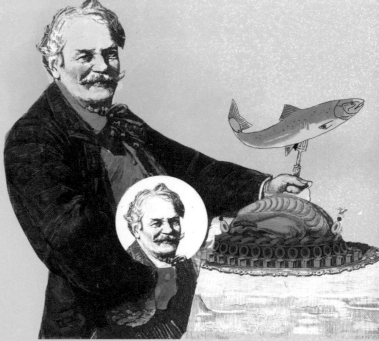

Happy tummy, happy head Anxiety and depression were thought to be an unchangeable and inherited weakness in the 18th and 19th centuries. Now experts are exploring how these mental illnesses can be treated by fostering healthy gut bacteria.

WHICH CAME FIRST?

Rodents specially bred to have no gut microbes (therefore germ-free) are used to help scientists study the gut microbiome. They have transferred the gut bacteria from anxious and depressed rats into healthy, germ-free rats to try and understand this relationship better. The scientists found that the healthy rodents took on depressed behaviors when they received the fecal transplant. One study even transferred bacteria from depressed people into germ-free rats and found the result to be the same.

There is also evidence that probiotics and antibiotics can change emotional behaviors (in rodents) by changing the microbiome. These studies all suggest that the bacteria in your gut can influence your state of mind.

Of course, it is not that straightforward. While some evidence shows that the microbiome affects mood, other evidence reveals that your mood, particularly stress and anxiety, affects your microbiome. Baby rats exposed to the stress of separation from their mothers undergo a change in their gut microbiome. When these baby rats were given probiotics, their stress

Bacteria do not physically travel between the gut and the brain. Instead they move via substances that make their way along a bi-directional pathway known as the microbe gut–brain axis (see pages 152–53).

levels went down. The gut–brain communication pathway appears to work in both directions.

GUT–BRAIN DISORDERS

The association between mood and the gut microbiome is causing scientists to view medical conditions such as IBS in a new light. People with IBS often suffer from depression or anxiety as well. The uncomfortable and often painful symptoms of the disease have frequently been blamed for mood changes associated with IBS, but now researchers are exploring whether the gut microbiome may also have a role to play. If so, treatments to promote "good" bacteria (see pages 112–13) and restore balance to the gut microbiome may not only alleviate the digestive symptoms of IBS, but also improve sufferers' mental health.

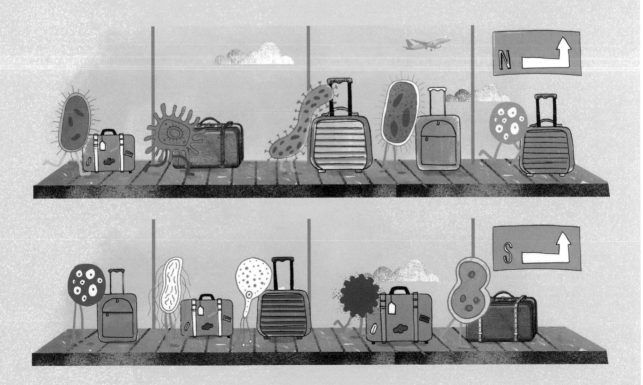

MICROBES AND THE GUT–BRAIN AXIS

In order to understand better how the gut microbiome affects mood and mental health, and vice versa, scientists are now examining the ways in which bacteria in the intestines communicate with the brain.

Your brain is a high-security area surrounded by the blood–brain barrier, which is designed to keep microbes and toxins out of the brain. Gut bacteria do not travel to the brain themselves. They either produce substances that are "approved" to cross this barrier or stimulate cells in the gut to do so. In other words, they tap into the body's existing systems (endocrine, neural and immune) that affect mood and mental health.

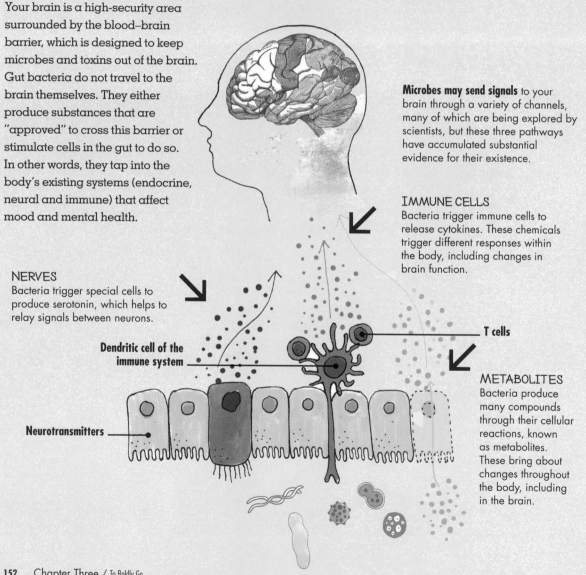

Microbes may send signals to your brain through a variety of channels, many of which are being explored by scientists, but these three pathways have accumulated substantial evidence for their existence.

IMMUNE CELLS
Bacteria trigger immune cells to release cytokines. These chemicals trigger different responses within the body, including changes in brain function.

NERVES
Bacteria trigger special cells to produce serotonin, which helps to relay signals between neurons.

T cells

Dendritic cell of the immune system

METABOLITES
Bacteria produce many compounds through their cellular reactions, known as metabolites. These bring about changes throughout the body, including in the brain.

Neurotransmitters

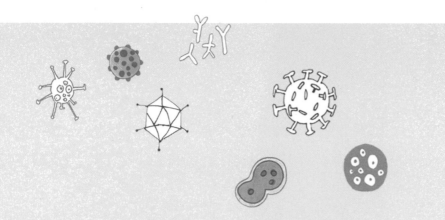

HIJACKING THE BODY'S COMMUNICATION SYSTEMS

Nerve cells: Bacteria produce substances that can trigger specialized cells in the gut to release neurotransmitters, such as serotonin. Serotonin itself cannot cross the blood–brain barrier, but it does stimulate the vagus nerve, which carries information from the gut to the brain. The stimulation is associated with improvements in mood, although more research is needed to understand why this is.

Immune cells: The mere presence of bacteria in the gut causes immune cells in the vicinity to release small proteins collectively known as cytokines. Their full role and functions are not yet understood, but cytokines can cross the blood–brain barrier and have both positive and negative effects within the body. For example, the good cytokines help the body to fight pathogens, while the bad cytokines have been linked to serious depression and inflammatory diseases, such as Crohn's disease. This may be one of the ways in which gut bacteria influence mood.

Metabolites: Most of the chemical substances that bacteria produce as they metabolize (such as the neurotransmitters serotonin and dopamine) are the same as those produced by your own cells. They therefore have the same effects within your body, including influencing mood.

Of all of these communication pathways, it is the stimulation of serotonin that has generated the most interest. This is because this neurotransmitter (known as the "feel-good" hormone) is so closely linked with mood and mental health. Around 90 percent of your serotonin is produced in the gut, making the gut's role critical in this respect.

Treatment: Considerable funding is now being directed toward understanding the gut–brain connection. The hope is that once more is known, the gut microbiome can be manipulated to improve mental health. For example, if certain strains of bacteria were discovered to produce metabolites that improved people's ability to deal with stress, or perhaps to make their bodies manufacture more serotonin, these might be encouraged — or even introduced into the gut through prebiotics and probiotics respectively. Until such treatments become established, sufficient evidence shows that people who eat a balanced diet — rich in fiber, fruits and vegetables — are less likely to suffer mental illness. So keep your digestion happy with good food, and you may also encourage a healthy mental state.

BEDTIME BUGS

Your mental health is closely linked to the quantity and quality of your sleep — people who suffer from anxiety or depression often have disrupted sleep patterns. Natural light levels, hormones and signals in the brain all affect your sleep, but gut bacteria can also play a part. They affect sleep indirectly by influencing your mood and anxiety levels, but they also produce
compounds that are important in regulating sleep cycles.

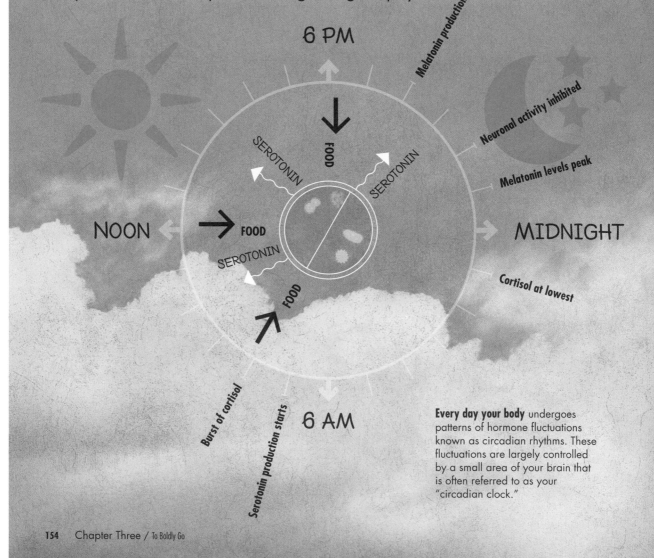

6 PM

Melatonin production

FOOD

SEROTONIN

SEROTONIN

Neuronal activity inhibited

Melatonin levels peak

NOON

FOOD

SEROTONIN

MIDNIGHT

FOOD

Cortisol at lowest

Burst of cortisol

Serotonin production starts

6 AM

Every day your body undergoes patterns of hormone fluctuations known as circadian rhythms. These fluctuations are largely controlled by a small area of your brain that is often referred to as your "circadian clock."

GUT MICROBES AND SLEEP

We still have a lot to learn about how the gut microbiome may influence sleep patterns. However, scientists do know that gut microbes stimulate the immune cells in your intestine to produce compounds that promote light sleep. During the day your body releases the hormone cortisol, which prevents these sleep compounds from being effective. As the day goes on cortisol levels drop, however, and sleep compounds start to take effect.

The gut microbiome can also affect sleep patterns by stimulating production of serotonin, the "happy hormone." As darkness falls, the low light levels prompt your body to start to convert serotonin into melatonin, the main sleep hormone. By stimulating serotonin production, the gut microbiome provides the foundations of a good night's sleep.

BACTERIAL RHYTHMS

The bacteria in your gut also have a daily rhythm. While you sleep, they perform several maintenance activities, such as getting rid of toxins that have accumulated within their cells and repairing DNA. When you wake up and start to eat, the bacteria spend more time growing, dividing and turning the food you have sent their way into energy.

The composition of your bacterial gut community also fluctuates over a 24-hour period. Certain species of bacteria are known to become more abundant at certain times of the day. There is even evidence that if you eat at a regular time each day, the beneficial *Lactobacillus reuteri* bacteria, involved in digestion, start to anticipate the arrival of food by expanding in numbers. They then offer protection from the bad bacteria you may consume by simply crowding them out.

DISRUPTED SLEEP PATTERNS

People who do shift work or who cross time zones frequently have their natural sleep patterns disrupted and tend to eat at irregular times. These disruptions can affect your gut microbiome as well, causing it to lose its daily rhythms. Sufferers from jet lag have higher numbers of species from the *Firmicutes* group of bacteria, which are linked to obesity and metabolic disease. There is limited evidence that these species die back once the person suffering from jet lag has recovered, but it is unclear what happens in the case of shift workers who change their sleep patterns frequently.

Disease-causing bacteria can survive for up to a week inside a plane. These microbial stowaways live in seat pockets, tray tables and armrests.

LIFESTYLE CHOICES AND OUR MICROBES

Sleep, mood and diet are not the only things that can affect (and be affected by) our bacteria. Your lifestyle shapes your microbiome: your hygiene habits, how much you drink, what you eat, whether you smoke and what activities you do all affect the community of bacteria that live in and on you in different ways.

Growing facial hair affects the bacterial community on the skin. A beard introduces new "resources" for bacteria and they are not disrupted daily by the act of shaving. Your choice of soap brand or type of clothing also affect the bacteria that live on you. Some of these subtler lifestyle differences might explain why two healthy people can have very different bacterial communities.

Although the human microbiome is relatively stable, many of our daily activities can have an immediate and substantial impact on the bacterial communities that call us home.

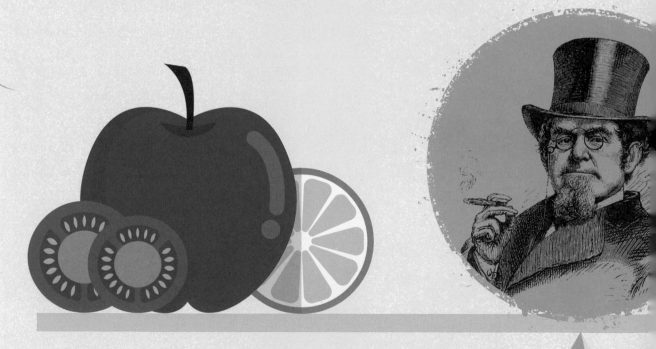

REGULAR EXERCISE

Exercise can increase both the number of beneficial bacteria and the diversity of species in your gut. It has a positive effect on mood and the brain, so exercise may indirectly affect gut microbes through the microbe gut–brain axis (see pages 152–53). But exercise also speeds up digestion, which may have a direct effect on your gut bacteria. It may favor species that are particularly efficient at harnessing energy from food before it moves through the colon.

ALCOHOL

Alcohol can slow the growth and the metabolism of bacteria — both good and bad — and yet many studies have shown that regular drinking can lead to a proliferation of bacteria in your intestinal tract. The problem is that these grow in areas where bacteria do not usually grow. Just one drink a day can lead to more bacteria than normal growing in your small intestine. Compared with the large intestine, the small intestine has relatively fewer bacteria, so a proliferation of this community can cause bloating, wind, abdominal pain, constipation or diarrhea.

For heavy drinkers, the situation is more serious. Continued heavy drinking results in bacteria crossing the gut lining and traveling through the bloodstream to the liver, which already works hard to remove alcohol from the blood. This organ then becomes a battleground for the immune system's attack on these bacterial intruders. This can cause permanent tissue damage in the liver, in addition to the tissue damage caused by the alcohol itself.

SMOKING

Cigarette smoke is a risk factor for many diseases. While the connection is obvious for some, such as lung cancer, others — for example inflammatory bowel diseases and Crohn's disease — are less clear. As changes in gut bacteria have also been linked to these diseases, scientists are trying to understand how smoking affects the human microbiome. A 2016 U.S. study found that the community of bacteria in the mouths of smokers was quite different than in those of non-smokers. Whether the bacterial communities associated with smokers can lead to disease is still being investigated.

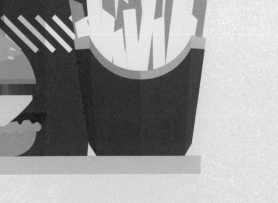

YOUR HEALTH HISTORY AND YOUR BUGS

The human microbiome is an ecosystem, vulnerable to disturbances. The illnesses you encounter, particularly in childhood, and their treatments affect this ecosystem. Your friendly bugs might be robust and bounce back after, say, a bout of diarrhea, but as with any ecosystem, repeated disturbances can lead to long-term consequences in the diversity of the species that live there.

Your health history can affect your friendly bacteria in several ways. They might be directly killed off by antibiotics taken to treat an illness or ejected from your body through the symptoms of your illness, such as diarrhea or substantial mucous production due to a cold. Your friendly bacteria might be directly affected by the introduction of a new organism, perhaps a parasite picked up on your travels or new bacteria introduced during a hospital stay. They may also be indirectly affected because an illness or accident changes the environment in which they live, for example the removal of an appendix or a severe burn to the skin.

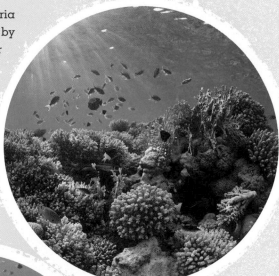

Repeated bouts of illness, such as norovirus, can have a similar effect on gut bacteria as repeated cyclones on a coral reef. The more frequent they are, the longer your bacteria take to recover their diversity (if ever).

ANTIBIOTICS

We expect antibiotics to affect good bacteria in the short term but longer term effects can also occur (see pages 46–47). These depend on the type of antibiotic used and the frequency and method of its administration. When scientists looked at the community of gut bacteria of people before and after taking the antibiotic clindamycin, they found that the beneficial *Bacteroides* species took two years to return to their pre-antibiotic numbers and diversity. When patients took the commonly used antibiotics for ulcer-causing *Helicobacter pylori* infections, some good gut bacteria species did not return until four years later.

Studies on children, whose microbiome is just developing, revealed that those treated with antibiotics within the first three years of life have less diverse and less stable communities of good bacteria in their guts than those not treated. Although they might have a similar number of species of good bacteria, they have fewer strains (see page 17). Their good bacteria have less genetic diversity, making it harder for them to adapt to changing situations. More research is needed to understand how long these differences in the microbiome last as children grow up.

REDUNDANT ORGANS

Recent research suggests the appendix, once thought a redundant organ, may act as a "safe house" for good bacteria in your gut. A bout of diarrhea caused by a gastrointestinal infection can effectively empty your intestines of friendly microbes. However, the appendix remains unaffected, so the good bacteria in the appendix can start to repopulate your gut as you recover.

Although the research has yet to be carried out, in theory the loss of the appendix may affect how well the gut microbiome bounces back after an illness; it may also determine which good bacteria recolonize the gut. There is evidence that people whose appendix is removed are more likely to suffer from colitis — an inflammation of the colon caused by the bacterium *Clostridium difficile*. Similarly, although research has yet to prove it, it is possible that people who have had their tonsils removed have a permanently altered oral microbiome as a result.

ANTIBIOTICS THAT END IN "MYCIN" COME FROM SUBSTANCES PRODUCED BY FUNGI

USING BUGS AS DRUGS

With evidence mounting that a diverse community of bacteria in your gut promotes good health, medical researchers are looking at different ways to encourage the growth of good bugs — not only to maintain good health, but also to treat conditions such as IBS and Crohn's disease. Prebiotics, probiotics and fecal transplant therapy are all ways of changing the microbiome for human health.

NOT JUST FOR YOUR GUT

Prebiotics and probiotics are not just for your gut. Ongoing research is looking at how topical prebiotics and probiotics may be helpful in skin health. In fact a species of bacteria found in natural hot springs, called *Vitreoscilla filiformis*, is thought to be the reason these natural spas have long been used to rejuvenate and treat inflammation of the skin. This species is now widely used in cosmetic products as a probiotic skin treatment.

POLY-BIOTICS ARE PROBIOTICS THAT CONTAIN MANY DIFFERENT STRAINS OF BACTERIA, A WHOLE BACTERIAL COMMUNITY IN A SACHET

SYNBIOTICS ARE PRODUCTS THAT CONTAIN BOTH PROBIOTICS AND PREBIOTICS

PREBIOTICS DELIVER THE NUTRIENTS THAT HELP GOOD BACTERIA TO THRIVE, WHILE PROBIOTICS DELIVER LIVE BACTERIA – IN OTHER WORDS, PREBIOTICS FEED PROBIOTICS

	PREBIOTICS	PROBIOTICS
What are they?	Indigestible fibre that is particularly nutritious to good bacteria, but not to bad bacteria	Live, good bacteria
How do they work?	Travel through your stomach and small intestine to the colon, where the good bacteria feed on them. Not harmed by the acidity of your stomach or your digestive enzymes	Travel through your stomach and small intestine to the colon; hopefully here they take up residence and multiply. Vulnerable to acidity and digestive enzymes, so not all of the ingested bacteria survive the trip to your colon
Natural sources	Foods such as artichokes, asparagus, bananas, garlic, leeks and onions	Yogurt, kefir, kimchi, kombucha, miso, sauerkraut and other fermented foods containing live cultures of bacteria (see page 162)
Other sources	Not all fibre is of equal nutritional value to your good bacteria (i.e. not all fibre is prebiotic). Manufacturers have isolated the most nutritious fibre for good bacteria and concentrated it into a dietary supplement (usually a powder or tablet; different brands use different recipes)	Many different brands of probiotics are available that contain different strains and combinations of species of live bacteria – usually in the form of an edible capsule
Pros	Supplements have a long shelf life and prebiotics are not affected by digestion, so what you eat always makes it to your colon	Probiotics can help to re-establish a diverse community of good bacteria in the gut after illness. Specific strains of bacteria can be taken if you are trying to promote the growth of particular bacteria
Cons	Prebiotics can only feed good bacteria if the latter are already present. It is not possible to promote the growth of a specific strain of good bacteria	Most of the probiotics you eat die before they reach your colon. Supplements can have a short shelf life and need refrigeration

BENEFICIAL BACTERIA

Humans have been using fermentation as a way of preserving food and making bread and alcohol for at least 7,000 years. The fermentation process first involves discouraging the growth of bad bacteria that will spoil the food by using heat or salt. Beneficial bacteria and/or yeasts are then added. These convert carbohydrates in the food into various products, including ethanol (wine and beer) and lactic acid (sauerkraut, kimchi and yogurt), as well as beneficial vitamins and fatty acids. Along with the nutritional benefits of fermented food, you get a good dose of these beneficial bacteria with every bite — they are natural probiotics.

Fermented foods such as cucumber pickles (made without vinegar), yogurt, kimchi, sauerkraut and kombucha all contain beneficial live bacteria.

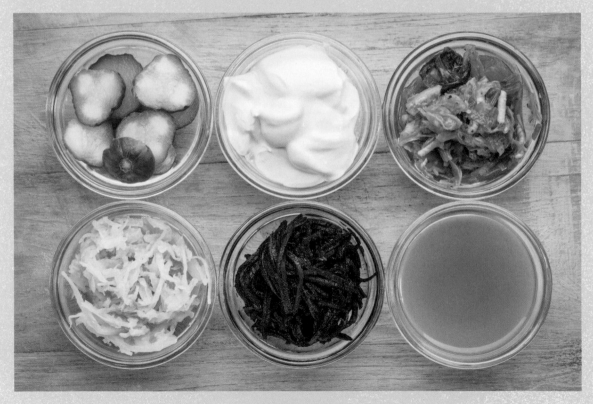

FECAL TRANSPLANTS

The procedure for fecal microbiota transplantation (FMT) is exactly as it sounds. Stool from a healthy donor is screened for bad bugs before being transferred to an unhealthy patient via a colonoscopy, enema or similar procedure. The advantage of a fecal transplant over probiotics or prebiotics is that it introduces a healthy community of bacteria directly to the area where it is needed, bypassing the stomach. Prebiotics may be given as well to encourage this new community to flourish.

The first documented cases of fecal transplants date back to China in the 4th-century AD, but they are currently gaining traction as a low-cost, low-risk treatment that is effective for a number of illnesses, including *Clostridium difficile* infections, IBS, Crohn's disease and ulcerative colitis. The challenge with fecal transplants is that they are hard to regulate — there is no consensus on the "ideal" microbiome so treatment cannot be standardized. However, stool banks are helping to formalize the process by screening donors and rigorously testing samples.

Stool banks collect feces from healthy donors just as blood banks do. In the U.S. donors can earn dollars for their donations.

MICROBIAL ECOSYSTEM THERAPEUTICS

Microbial ecosystem therapy (MET) takes fecal transplants one step further. A sample from a healthy donor is meticulously screened for any less desirable bugs, including good bacteria that have acquired antibiotic resistance. Beneficial bacteria are isolated from the healthy stool sample and these are added to a community of other known beneficial bacteria, the idea being that bacteria are happiest when in a diverse community. This concoction, nicknamed "RePOOPulate" by the Canadian researchers pioneering the method, is then transplanted into the patient via a colonoscopy. The advantage of this method is that it gives researchers a little more control over the bacterial community being transplanted. This results in greater potential for standardizing or indeed modifying the community to cure specific ailments as scientists learn more about the human microbiome and disease.

163

STERILE ENVIRONMENTS

Sterile environments and techniques can be vital — surgical instruments in an operating room, for example — but is our concern with killing germs in daily life too great? The use of anti-bacterial soaps, sanitizers and cleaning equipment has implications for the environment. They may also have created unnaturally sterile environments with consequences for human health.

The sterile environments created in homes and offices are thought to be one of the main reasons for the increase in allergies among people of developed countries. Frequent exposure to good bacteria in the environment, particularly as a child, is important for the development of the immune system and maintaining equilibrium in the body (homeostasis, see page 36).

Wiping down worktops regularly with harsh cleaning agents (rather than just in the area of a spill) removes the layer of harmless bacteria that live there. These would otherwise help to keep bad bacteria in check by outcompeting bad bacteria for resources.

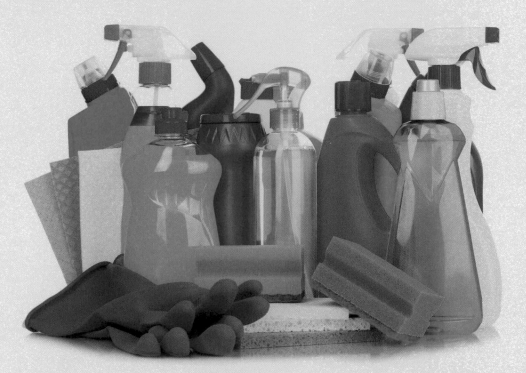

THE HYGIENE HYPOTHESIS

This theory suggests that insufficient exposure as a young child to bacteria, both good and bad, prevents the immune system from developing normally. As a result an older child may become less tolerant of harmless substances such as pollen or dust. The presence of siblings and pets is likely to expose children to more bacteria. A busy household might also mean less time being spent on housework, and therefore a less sterile environment. The constant exposure to bacteria, as well as other microbes, enables the developing immune system to fine-tune its discernment of good bacteria from bad.

GOOD HYGIENE

While the hygiene hypothesis sounds like a useful excuse to shirk housework, some areas of the home do require very good hygiene. For example, chopping boards used for cutting raw meat, particularly chicken, should be washed immediately, while those used for vegetables can be washed later. Using separate chopping boards for meat and vegetables is also advised. Environments that are warm and damp allow both good and bad bacteria to proliferate, so kitchen towels, for example, should be replaced daily. Do not rinse raw chicken under the tap when preparing it — bacteria on its surface can be carried in the water droplets, which are then sprayed around kitchen surfaces. On the same basis, close the toilet lid before flushing to prevent bacteria in the swirling water and waste spraying out onto anything nearby.

PROBIOTIC CLEANERS

Probiotic cleaners containing beneficial bacteria rather than antibacterial chemicals are now available on the market. They work on the same principle as consuming probiotices to influence the the human microbiome (see pages 160–61): by covering surfaces with a community of good bacteria, the good bacteria can outcompete the bad.

There is also evidence that chemical-based cleaners may contribute to the development of drug-resistant strains of bacteria, so probiotic cleaners are being considered for hospital use. Italian researchers who developed a cleaner containing the spores of harmless *Bacillus* species found that it reduced the number of pathogenic bacteria on hospital surfaces by as much as 90 percent more than conventional disinfectants. Nor did it encourage the development of resistant strains.

COMPUTER KEYBOARDS CAN BE MATCHED UP WITH THEIR OWNERS BY IDENTIFYING THE BACTERIAL COMMUNITIES FOUND ON BOTH

METROPOLITAN MICROBES, COUNTRY CRITTERS

If you live in an urban environment, the bacteria inhabiting your home are mostly species from your body — bacteria from your skin, mouth and gut. However, if you live in a more rural environment, a far bigger proportion of the bacteria in your home come from outside — soil and air. These differences in bacteria may explain why city dwellers sometimes contract different diseases from those living in the country.

Although each city has its own identifiable bacterial community, they are not as distinctive as the bacterial communities found in rural areas. This is probably because cities have a greater migration of people.

WHY SO DIFFERENT?

The differences in these bacterial communities are fundamentally based on the extent to which the inside and outside environments interact, along with the nature of the latter. A tenth-floor apartment with two opening windows, for example, will have far less air exchange than a country house with windows on all sides, where air is allowed to flow through. The bacteria brought into the home on shoes and clothes from a farm, muddy fields or woodland are very different from those brought in from a city street. Even something as simple as using freshly dug carrots caked in dirt or plastic-wrapped carrots from the supermarket affects what types of bacteria inhabit the home.

HUMAN SKIN BACTERIA ACCOUNT FOR AROUND 30 PERCENT OF THE BACTERIA FOUND IN AN OFFICE

URBAN VS RURAL GUT MICROBIOME

The different bacterial communities found in urban and rural environments also impact the human microbiome. While you might expect this to be because the bacteria in the environment differ, it seems also to be related to differences in diet. A study in Russia, for example, revealed that the microbiomes of Russian city dwellers resembled Western cultures more than those of rural Russians. Scientists suspect this is due to the more Western lifestyles that Russians in urban settings lead, including the greater consumption of meat and processed food. More research is needed to understand these differences and what they may mean for human health.

HUMAN HEALTH

In statistical terms children in the country develop fewer allergies and less asthma. In part this is because they are exposed to more and different bacteria in their environment than children in cities. However, it is still unclear how the different bacterial communities of urban and rural settings impact human health overall. Other health-related factors, including socio-economic status, access to healthcare and local air quality, also contribute to people's well-being.

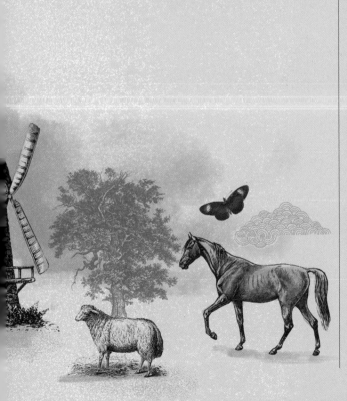

BACTERIA IN BUILDINGS

Within the same city, different buildings have their own bacterial communities. Even within a building, however, the bacterial communities differ from room to room. A bathroom contains bacteria associated with the human gut, while those in a bedroom are associated with skin. The two main factors that affect the types of bacteria occupying a building seem to be related to how it is ventilated and who occupies it.

The number of people occupying a room, the amount of time they spend there and whether it is the same group of people every day or a different set all affect a room's microbiome.

The more interconnected indoor spaces are, through open-concept layouts or multiple doors, the more similar the bacterial communities in these areas will be.

PRESCHOOLS

In a preschool environment germs spread rapidly: toys are chewed, small hands wipe runny noses and then pick up a crayon, and so on. As a result, children in nurseries are three to four times more likely to have a respiratory infection than those kept at home. But, according to the hygiene hypothesis (see page 97), this is valuable training for children's immune systems. The thinking around preschool facilities is therefore slowly shifting from preventing the spread of germs — which would be impossible —

Rooms ventilated by open windows contain higher numbers of bacteria associated with soil and plants than those ventilated by filtered ventilation systems.

to spreading the right germs. Disinfectants are increasingly only recommended for targeting those places where harmful bacteria might thrive, such as toilets or where a child has been ill, rather than throughout school facilities. Avoiding the widespread use of these harmful chemicals is now thought to be better for the children, the environment and possibly the classroom's microbiome.

CARE HOMES

Care homes house people who are often more vulnerable to infections and may frequently be prescribed antibiotics. Consequently, care workers must take precautions to avoid spreading infectious diseases between the people in their charge, while also encouraging good bacteria in the facility that might outcompete the bad. Research has shown that rooms ventilated with fresh air contain fewer bacteria that cause diseases in humans, and designs for new care homes and hospitals are starting to reflect this knowledge, albeit slowly. Perhaps in the future architects will design for healthy bugs as well as patients.

BACTERIAL BUILDING INSPECTIONS?

Some scientists have speculated that in the future we may pay greater attention to the bacteria associated with a building. Just as buildings have different eco-certifications to determine their sustainability in terms of materials sourced and energy used, there may also be microbiome certifications that rank a building's bacteria-friendly features. Perhaps in the future potential purchasers will even hire inspectors to check a home's microbiome before buying?

ANTIBIOTICS IN AGRICULTURE

In the 1950s farmers started to raise animals in smaller spaces, to derive more product from less land. But disease spreads quickly in such conditions. To counter this, the agricultural industry began to add antibiotics to animal feed as a preventative measure, even if the animals were not sick. They found that not only did the crowded animals fall ill less often, but they grew faster, thereby improving profits. This is known as non-therapeutic antibiotic treatment.

Resistant bacteria, which develop on farms through routine use of antibiotics, can be transferred in the following ways:

(1) Between animals on the farm.

(2) In animal waste, which is then spread on fields and can pass into the soil or onto growing crops.

(3) In animal waste, which leaches out into nearby streams. Here resistance can get passed onto aquatic bacteria or bacteria associated with aquatic life, such as fish.

(4) Between farm workers and others, or through contaminated products sold by the farmer.

(5) These various pathways may eventually lead to the general population, although far away from the farm itself, and in turn cause difficult-to-treat bacterial infections.

Global concerns over the emergence of antibiotic-resistant strains of bacteria have forced governments to reduce the non-therapeutic use of antibiotics. In 1986 Sweden became the first country to ban their use, and many other countries have since followed suit. Countries such as the U.S., however, still allow their use. It is estimated that in 2012 some 80 percent of the antimicrobial drugs sold in the U.S. (by weight) were for animals, and that 60 percent of those drugs were also used in human medicine. Resistance developed on farms therefore has serious implications for human health.

SPREADING

When bacteria are constantly exposed to an antibiotic, it creates a stressful situation that triggers them to adapt to this new environment. Mutations evolve that help the bacteria to survive under these conditions (see pages 30–31). There are many different ways in which bacteria can resist an antibiotic — the bacterium can produce an enzyme that destroys the drug, for example, or coat itself in a capsule that the antibiotic is unable to penetrate. Because there are several different types of resistance, these are collectively called the resistance factor (or R-factor). The resistant bacteria thrive; they pass on the resistance factor to their progeny, as well as to other bacteria — even possibly those outside their species — through conjugation, transduction or transformation (see pages 28–29).

IMPLICATIONS FOR HUMAN HEALTH

The link between the overuse of antibiotics in agriculture and antibiotic-resistant bacteria affecting humans has been made many times over. Resistant bacteria have been traced back to meat grown on farms where growth-promoting bacteria are being used. In 1999 the European Union banned the non-therapeutic agricultural use of any antibiotics employed in human medicine. Seven years later the European Union banned the non-therapeutic use of antibiotics in agriculture altogether.

The incidence of disease in agriculture can be reduced by keeping animals under appropriate conditions, in lower densities and in clean facilities. After the ban of these non-therapeutic antibiotics, many countries recorded lower agricultural productivity, but this seemed a small price to pay compared to creating difficult-to-treat bacteria that posed a serious threat to human health. In countries such as the U.K., where antibiotics are banned for non-therapeutic purposes, they are still prescribed by veterinarians to treat sick animals. But, just as the attitude toward prescribing antibiotics in human healthcare has changed over the decades, so has the use of antibiotics in agriculture.

IT IS ESTIMATED THAT LIVESTOCK IN THE U.S. ARE GIVEN 29 MILLION POUNDS OF ANTIBIOTICS EVERY YEAR

SUPERBUGS EXPOSED

In hospitals, where antibiotics are widely used and disease-causing bacteria lurk, resistance factors are unfortunately common. Bacteria excel at passing resistance factors between each other and when they acquire several of these factors, they transform into superbugs, which pose a serious threat to humans.

Hospital environments, where antibiotics are in constant use for treating and preventing infections, speed up the evolution of antibiotic resistance in bacteria, just as agriculture has done (see pages 170–71). Despite best efforts to keep things sterile, these resistant bacteria migrate around the hospital on both equipment and people. Some are able to pick up multiple resistance factors and so become "superbugs." The development of superbugs is a global problem: resistance can spread rapidly as people and products constantly circulate around the planet. There is growing concern that infectious diseases may not be controllable in the near future, as the antibiotics currently available are ineffective against these superbugs.

Carbapenem-resistant Enterobacteriaceae

Helicobacter pylori

Superbugs have acquired several resistance factors, which make them resistant to multiple antibiotics.

Mycobacterium tuberculosis

MULTIDRUG-RESISTANT TUBERCULOSIS (MDR-TB)

Tuberculosis causes approximately 1.8 million deaths each year, making it the number one killer among infectious diseases. About 250,000 of these deaths are caused by a drug-resistant strain of *Mycobacterium tuberculosis*. To try and combat multidrug-resistant tuberculosis, patients are given a very complex and long-term treatment (lasting 6–24 months) of several less effective medicines; these take a toll on the body and are only successful half of the time. Some strains of *Mycobacterium* have even become resistant to these second-line treatments. These are known as extensively drug-resistant strains, and only one-third of patients infected with such strains are treated successfully. There have only been two new antibiotic treatments found for MDR-TB in the last 70 years. This lack of treatment combined with the prevalence of the disease make finding new treatments for MDR-TB a global priority.

CARBAPENEM-RESISTANT ENTEROBACTERIACEAE (CRE)

The second most concerning group of superbugs belong to a family of bacteria known as *Enterobacteriaceae*. This family includes familiar groups such as *Salmonella*, *Escherichia coli* and *Yersinia pestis*. They have developed resistance to carbapenem antibiotics, a group of "last ditch" antibiotics used to treat patients who are hospitalized with multidrug-resistant bacterial infections. Bacteria from the *Enterobacteriaceae* family produce an enzyme that breaks down the antibiotics, and approximately 50 percent of people with a CRE infection die.

AVOIDING SUPERBUGS

Everyone is susceptible to an infection by a superbug. The following may help to reduce your risk of exposure:

- Take precautions when around people with an infection: wash hands thoroughly and avoid sharing cups or food, or personal items such as razors or toothbrushes

- Keep healthy, in order to avoid a stay in hospital where superbugs lurk, and benefit from a stronger immune system

- Prepare food safely: wash your hands, wash fruit and vegetables, cook food at the right temperature, use separate chopping boards for raw and ready-to-eat food (salad, fruit), store raw meat and fish in separate containers at the bottom of the fridge

- Limit antibiotics: most health professionals avoid prescribing antibiotics unless absolutely necessary, but if offered a prescription, ask whether it is critical that you take it

- Be cautious while traveling: in some countries the use of growth-promoting antibiotics in agriculture, combined with less stringent food safety regulations, unclean water and lack of sanitation, can increase the likelihood of antibiotic-resistant bacteria spreading. Also bear this in mind if considering "medical tourism"

- Seek medical advice quickly: there is a better chance of curing an infection if caught early

ANTIBIOTICS ON THE HORIZON

As more antibiotics become ineffective against bacteria, there are broader implications for healthcare. Major surgeries and medical treatments such as cesarean sections, heart surgery or hip replacements, cancer chemotherapy, organ transplants and diabetes management all become very high risk without antibiotics to prevent bacterial infections. New antibiotics are urgently needed.

LOOKING FOR NEW ANTIBIOTICS

Scientists have found potential candidates for the development of new antibiotic drugs in surprising places. Researchers at the University of Nottingham studied cockroaches, well known for surviving in all sorts of (often filthy) conditions. They discovered that a substance in the cockroach's brain seems to be particularly effective at killing *E. coli*, which causes bacterial meningitis, and MRSA.

In their search for new antibiotics, scientists often look to plants and animals that spend a lot of time in "dirty" places or are known to produce other interesting chemical substances.

Other scientists turned their attention to fish due to the antimicrobial substances in the mucous that coats their skin and scales. The catfish, which spends most of its time sitting in the muddy, bacteria-rich sediments of freshwater lakes and slow-moving rivers, is a perfect candidate. One substance isolated from catfish seems to be very good at killing *Klebsiella pneumoniae*, which can sometimes cause pneumonia as well as urinary tract infections.

A bacterial species found living in the sediments on the floor of the Pacific Ocean has been of considerable interest over the last few years. It produces an antibiotic effective against anthrax, an infection caused by *Bacillus anthracis*, as well as MRSA, but research is still in the exploratory phase.

The many interesting substances produced by the cannabis plant (cannabinoids) are being explored for their antibiotic properties and for a host of medicinal purposes, from the treatment of seizures to cancer.

SCIENTISTS HAVE IDENTIFIED 100 POTENTIAL ANTIBIOTIC SUBSTANCES FROM EXAMINING THE SKIN OF 6,000 DIFFERENT FROG SPECIES

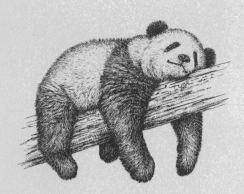

Panda bears are also of interest due to the antibiotic substance in their blood that takes a fraction of the time to kill bacteria compared with some commonly used antibiotics (one-sixth to be exact).

FUNDING THE SEARCH

Although the need for new antibiotics is clear, there has until recently been a lack of funding for such research. This is largely because pharmaceutical companies know that newly developed antibiotics will be dished out only sparingly to minimize the formation of resistant strains of bacteria.

To make research funds stretch further, scientists have been examining existing drugs for potential antibiotic properties. In 2017 findings were published stating that long-term users of statins — a group of medicines used to lower cholesterol — were less likely to suffer *Staphylococcus aureus* infections. New antibiotics can come from anywhere, including well-established drugs.

Also in 2017 the World Health Organization's Global Antibiotic R&D Partnership announced $69 million in funding to fight antibiotic resistance, including searching for new antibiotics. The U.S. Government also announced a $62 million contract to conduct final testing of a novel antibiotic called ridinilazole. Developed by a U.K. biotech firm, this antibiotic may be useful in treating *Clostridium difficile* infections.

VACCINES

An alternative to fighting infections with antibiotics is to prime your immune system, so that when it encounters bad bacteria it launches immediately into a full attack. This is exactly what vaccines do. They provide your immune system with memories of some very bad bacteria, rather like posting "wanted" posters all over town.

B cells retain a memory of that bacteria. They will produce antibodies immediately if and when they encounter it, should you become infected.

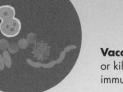

Vaccines contain weakened or killed bacterial cells, which the immune system attacks.

TYPES OF VACCINES

If a vaccine is not strong enough, your immune system will respond weakly, not necessarily building a memory against the bad bacteria for the future, so when scientists are developing a vaccine they need to achieve the right balance. The vaccine needs to be strong enough to prompt a response from the immune system so that it builds a memory against the bad bacteria for the future. However, it can't be so strong that it makes someone ill. Certain types of vaccines are better at this than others depending on the pathogen.

Some vaccines contain whole cells of bacteria that have been killed (inactivated) or weakened (attenuated) in some way. The vaccine for whooping cough, for example, contains dead whole-cells of the bacterium responsible, *Bordetella pertussis*. The vaccine Ty21a for typhoid fever, on the other hand, contains live cells of *Salmonella typhi*, but they have been chemically weakened.

Toxoid vaccines do not contain a weakened version of the bacteria themselves, just the toxins they produce. DTaP vaccine contains the weakened toxins of the bacteria species *Clostridium tetani and Corynebacterium diphtheriae*, which cause tetanus and diphtheria respectively. Other vaccines, known as subunit vaccines, contain only parts of the bacteria — usually specific proteins. These create an immune response sufficient that if and when your immune system encounters the whole bacteria, it will recognize that one part and attack. However, these vaccines tend to be expensive as it takes a lot of time (and therefore money) for researchers to identify which parts of the bacteria evoke the best response from the immune system.

The last type of vaccine uses a closely related species of bacterium — one that your immune system reacts to but that does not cause disease in humans. This vaccine has to be close enough to the human pathogen to be useful. *Mycobacterium bovis*, which causes tuberculosis in cattle, is used to protect humans against the tuberculosis-causing bacterium *Mycobacterium tuberculosis*.

Depending on the vaccine, the immune system often needs more than one dose in order to develop a sufficiently strong memory against the bad bacteria. The immune system may also start to lose its memory if not exposed to the bad bacteria for a long time. "Booster" vaccinations — for tetanus, for example — are given to "remind" the immune system about the bad bacteria.

PROTECT YOUR NEIGHBORS

Some people cannot be vaccinated against certain diseases due to their age or health conditions. However, if 80 percent of the population around them is vaccinated, the disease is unable to spread easily through the population, reducing the risk to those who are not vaccinated — a situation known as "herd immunity." If only some of the population is immunized, however, herd immunity starts to break down. This becomes particularly important in the face of antimicrobial resistance. With fewer options for treating an infection, the best defense for many might be a strong attack — vaccination.

NANOTECHNOLOGY AND SUPERBUGS

There are 1,000 nanometers in a single micrometer (micron), so while a bacterium that is a micron in diameter might seem small, a nanoparticle is tiny by comparison. This means that nanoparticles can be powerful tools in the fight against bad bacteria.

When particles are reduced to the nanoscale, their physical and chemical properties change. Iron, for example, becomes so reactive it can be used to remove arsenic from water and clean up contaminated land. This is because nanoparticles have a greater surface area with which to react. For example, a cube measuring 1in × 1in × 1in has a surface area of 6 in^2 (6 sides, 1in^2 each). However, if you were to fill that same volume with nanocubes measuring 1nm × 1nm × 1nm each, the combined surface area of all those nanocubes would be 9,000,183.6 in^2. (A 1 centimeter cube would result in a surface area of 60 million cm^2.)

Nano-sized particles come into contact with far more of the cell surface of a bacterium than larger micron-sized particles.

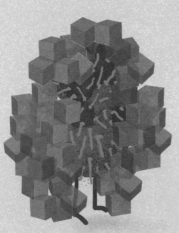

THERE IS NANOSILVER IN YOUR UNDERWEAR! IT HAS ANTIBACTERIAL PROPERTIES SO IT IS USED IN ALL TYPES OF CLOTHING

HOW IT WORKS

Scientists have identified a whole list of ways in which nanoparticles do harm to bacteria. The details are still being worked out, but, much like antibiotics, nanoparticles disrupt the growth or reproduction of the bacterial cells in some way. Nanosilver, for example, physically damages the cell, anchoring to the cell membrane and penetrating it, breaking the cell open. Nanoparticles of other materials, such as titanium oxide, release highly reactive oxygen (free radicals), which chemically damages the bacterium's cell membrane. Other nanoparticles block cell functions, such as protein synthesis, within the bacterium and so kill it. And some nanoparticles even incorporate themselves into the bacterial DNA and mess up the "recipe book" directly (see page 30).

DRUG DELIVERY SERVICE

Nanotechnology is also being used to deliver antibiotics directly to superbugs. A nanoparticle coating can protect the drug from breaking down in the body too quickly or make it more soluble. The nanoparticle capsules can even be designed to break open only when they experience a certain pH. This could be used to deliver a drug safely past the acidity of the stomach in order to target bad bacteria in the intestine.

BIODEGRADABLE NANO-NINJAS

Scientists in the U.S. have been developing "ninja polymers," a potential new weapon against antibiotic-resistant bacteria. Nanostructures self-assemble upon contact with water, joining together to form a more powerful structure – the ninja polymer. Scientists are able to design the ninja polymers to have a positive electric charge so that they seek out the strongly negative-charged cells infected with bad bacteria. The ninja polymer then attaches to the cell's surface and ruptures the membrane, killing the infected cell as well as the bacteria. The nano-sized ninja polymers are then naturally destroyed by the body's own enzymes, degrading them into particles that can either be broken down further or removed as waste.

The nano-ninjas were originally developed by scientists at IBM for building computer chips.

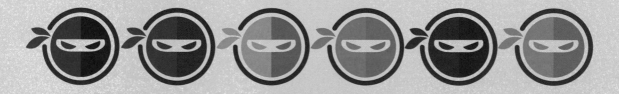

BUGS THROUGH THE AGES

Human lifestyles have altered dramatically throughout our evolution, from hunter-gatherers to agriculturalists, and on through industrialization to the globalization we know today. These developments have lead to fundamental changes to what we eat, the environments we spend time in and who we spend time with — all of which impact the human microbiome.

Humans have been evolving, along with their bacteria, since before we first began to stand upright. Knowledge of the ancestral microbiome can provide an important context for our understanding of the microbiome of the modern healthy human being.

The soft tissue of frozen mummified humans, such as the Tyrolean iceman known as Ötzi who lived between around 3400 and 3100 BC, contains bacterial DNA. This can help scientists understand which bacteria were part of the microbiome of ancient peoples.

DESICCATED OR FOSSILIZED FECES ARE ANOTHER SOURCE OF ANCIENT BACTERIA

A GLIMPSE INTO THE PAST

Scientists analyzing the gut bacteria of traditional hunter-gatherer societies have discovered they had a much more diverse community of gut bacteria than those with a diet based on modern agriculture.

These hunter-gatherer societies provide a window into what the human microbiome might have looked like before agriculture. Intrigued by such differences in diversity, the scientists explored the question further using mice. They found that a less varied diet for mice led to a less diverse community of gut bacteria, which could be reversed by expanding the variation in the diet again. However, if they did not expand the diversity of the diet again until the fourth generation of mice, the diversity of gut bacteria never recovered. Such a discovery has led scientists to speculate that the progressively narrowed diet we eat as humans is irreversibly changing the diversity of our gut bacteria.

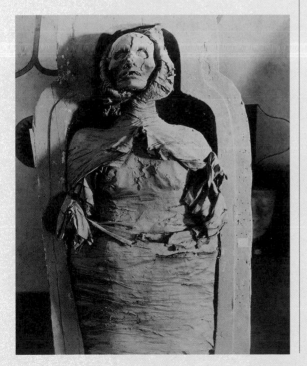

LEARNING FROM ANCIENT BUGS

Scientists have gleaned numerous insights from looking at ancient bugs found in mummified bodies and fossilized stools:

- Bacteria in the human microbiome developed antibiotic-resistant genes before antibiotics were used for the treatment of disease

- The bacterium *Streptococcus mutans*, which causes tooth decay, became far more wide-spread at around the time that humans adopted an agricultural lifestyle

- Many of the same bacteria — good and bad — linked to humans today have been associated with humans for millennia

- The diversity of human gut bacteria has reduced rapidly throughout the evolution of modern humans, possibly related to the fact that we cook our food

- The bacteria found in ancient humans, such as the Tyrolean iceman, are more closely aligned to the modern microbiomes of people living in rural than in urban environments

Together with these new insights, scientists are also using their new found knowledge of our ancestors' ancient bacterial passengers to help trace human migration routes. The spread of bacteria can illustrate how different peoples moved across the land to colonize new areas.

Studies of mummified ancient Egyptians have revealed that many may have died from bacterial diseases with which we are familiar today, including tuberculosis, caused by Mycobacterium tuberculosis.

GLOBAL BACTERIA

Since your bacteria are ultimately sourced from your immediate environment, it is not surprising that where you live has a powerful effect on your personal bacteria community. While each person's individual microbiome is unique, those of people living in the same area will share similarities. Global differences in the microbiome may explain why certain diseases are more prevalent in some parts of the world than in others.

A major study carried out in 2012 examined the gut flora of more than 500 people living in countries as diverse as the U.S., Venezuela (South America) and Malawi (Africa). The results were striking. Despite the distance between them, the microbiomes of people in Venezuela and Malawi were more similar to each other than to the microbiomes of those in the U.S.. Other studies have also confirmed this distinction in microbiomes between inhabitants of developing countries and developed countries, indicating that geographical differences in the microbiome are also driven by diet, lifestyle and culture.

WHAT WE EAT

Many studies conclude that it is more about what you eat than where you eat. Remote hunter-gatherer communities around the world share more similarities in their gut microbiomes than with their neighboring farming or urban populations, for example. Remote hunter-gatherers have a very high diversity of bacteria with enriched numbers of *Prevotella*, *Treponema* and *Succinovibrio*, and might suffer from intestinal parasites, but diseases such as Type 2 diabetes and autoimmune diseases are unheard of. Urban industrialized populations have low bacterial diversity and, while they do not have intestinal parasites, they suffer from many diseases associated with the gut microbiome, such as IBS and Type 2 diabetes. Traditional farming and fishing communities lie somewhere between these two extremes.

WHAT WE DO

Geographical differences in the skin microbiome appear to be related to cultural behaviors. A comparison of the skin microbiome between the hands of women living in the U.S. and those in Tanzania revealed a far higher prevalence of species associated with soil on the hands of the latter. Tanzanian women spend more time outdoors and activities such as cooking are often performed on the ground. There also seems to be a loss of diversity in skin bacteria as people move from nomadic lifestyles, in which they are more exposed to the environment, to living in permanent houses.

WHO WE ARE

Host genetics also affect the human microbiome. Your microbiome is more similar to that of your family than it is to non-family members, though it is difficult to know whether this is due to nature or nurture. However, a study of identical and non-identical twins found that the microbiomes of identical twins are far closer than those of non-identical twins, suggesting that there is a genetic component at play here.

A study of 1,000 twins in the U.K. confirmed that the host genotype helps to shape which species of bacteria colonize the microbiome.

GLOSSARY

AEROBIC BACTERIA Bacteria that require oxygen to live and grow.

ALLERGY An overreaction by the immune system to a usually harmless substance (such as pollen or a foodstuff) that results in symptoms ranging from sneezing or skin rashes to severe breathing difficulties.

AMINO ACIDS The building blocks of proteins. Of the 21 amino acids in humans, around half cannot be made by the human body and need to come from our diets.

ANAEROBIC BACTERIA Bacteria that can live and grow in the absence of oxygen.

ANTIBIOTIC A medicine that can inhibit the growth of or destroy bacteria.

ANTIBODY A specialized protein of the immune system produced by B cells. Antibodies help the immune system to destroy harmful bacteria or viruses.

ANTIOXIDANT A substance that helps to prevent cell damage caused by the free radicals generated by oxygen metabolism.

ARCHAEA Small, single-celled microorganisms that resemble bacteria but with some structural differences.

AUTOIMMUNE DISEASE A disease in which the immune system reacts inappropriately, attacking and damaging the body's own tissues.

BACTERIOPHAGE A virus that infects and destroys bacteria.

BACTERIUM A member of a large group of single-celled prokaryotic microorganisms, with cell walls but no nucleus.

B CELL A key lymphocyte (white blood cell) of the immune system. With the help of T cells, they make specific antibodies against bacteria and viruses.

BIOFILM A thin layer of bacterial cells, adhering to a surface and encased in a protective coating, making the bacteria more resistant to disinfectants and antibiotics.

CAPSULE A gelatinous layer that forms part of the outer envelope of some bacterial cells.

CHROMOSOME A thread-like strand of protein and DNA in the cell nucleus. Chromosomes carry genetic information in the form of genes.

CLONE The daughter cell that comes from a single bacterium dividing through fission. It is genetically identical to the original cell.

COLONY A visible mass of bacteria derived from a single mother cell and therefore are genetically identical (clones).

COMMENSALISM A relationship between two kinds of organisms in which one obtains food or other benefits from the other, without damaging or benefitting it.

COMMUNITY Groups of bacteria from different species that live together in the same place.

CONJUGATION The transfer of genetic material between bacterial cells by cell-to-cell contact or by a bridge-like connection between two cells.

CYTOKINES A large group of proteins, mainly secreted by cells of the immune system. Cytokines affect the behavior of numerous different types of cell that they encounter. They play a particular role in regulating immune responses, in both positive and negative ways.

CYTOPLASM The jelly-like fluid that surrounds the nucleus to fill a living cell.

DNA Genetic material contained in chromosomes found in the nucleus of most cells. A section of DNA with the genetic code for making a particular protein is called a gene.

DOPAMINE An important neurotransmitter (messenger) in the brain, which helps regulate emotion and movement.

ENTEROTYPE In a similar way to blood group classification, people can be grouped by the types of bacteria in their gut.

ENZYME A biological catalyst — a substance that speeds up chemical reactions but remains unchanged itself.

EPITHELIUM One or more layers of densely packed cells that form a thin covering, such as on the outer layer (epidermis) of the skin or a lining on the inside of the gut.

EUKARYOTE A cell or organism with a membrane-bound nucleus containing its genetic material (DNA). Animals, plants and fungi are eukaryotes.

FECAL TRANSPLANT Also fecal microbiota transplantation (FMT). Good bacteria from a healthy donor are transplanted into the gut of another person lacking certain essential bacteria.

FERMENTATION The process by which a complex substance is chemically broken down into a simpler substance, usually by microorganisms such as yeast or bacteria.

FISSION The process in which one cell splits into two new identical daughter cells. Bacteria reproduce asexually, by binary fission.

FLAGELLUM A microscopic, tail-like structure that projects from a bacterial cell. It enables the bacterium to move around.

FREE RADICALS Toxic by-products of oxygen metabolism that can cause significant damage to living cells and tissues.

GENOME The complete set of genetic material in an organism.

GRAM-POSITIVE/-NEGATIVE Gram-positive bacteria are those more receptive to antibiotics than gram-negative bacteria. The latter have a more resistant cell wall.

GRANULOCYTE A white blood cell that contains small granules. Granulocytes help the immune system to fight off viruses and bacteria.

GUT FLORA The resident bacteria in the gut.

GUT LUMEN The channel inside the gut along which food moves.

HISTAMINE A compound released by cells in response to injury and in allergic reactions, causing inflammation and swelling.

HOMEOSTASIS The regulation of conditions in the body, such as temperature and carbon dioxide levels. Such regulation ensures that the body's different systems are kept in check and conditions remain relatively constant.

HORMONE A chemical messenger that helps to regulate processes in the body. Hormones are secreted by a range of glands in the body and travel to their target organ or tissues in the bloodstream.

IMMUNE SYSTEM The cells (including white blood cells), tissues and organs (lymph nodes, spleen and thymus) that work together to protect the body from pathogens (viruses, parasites and bacteria) and other foreign substances.

LYMPHATIC SYSTEM A circulatory system connected by lymphatics (thin tubes), comprising bone marrow, thymus, spleen and lymph nodes (where immune cells are "trained"). The system transports immune cells around the body in a clear fluid called lymph.

MACROPHAGE A large white blood cell that occurs in tissues, particularly at sites of infection, or in the bloodstream. It engulfs and destroys microorganisms, such as bacteria.

MAST CELL An immune cell commonly found beneath the skin surface and throughout the respiratory, urinary and digestive systems. The cell releases histamines and other molecules during inflammatory and allergic reactions.

METABOLISM The chemical processes that occur within a living organism, such as a bacterium, in order to maintain life.

METABOLITE A substance formed by, or necessary for, metabolism.

MICROBE A bacterium, in particular one that causes disease. Microbe is often used interchangeably with microorganism.

MICROBIOME All the microorganisms in a particular environment, for example the human body.

MICRON Also called a micrometer. Symbol μm. 1 μm = 0.001 mm and approximately 0.000039 inch.

MICROORGANISM A microscopic organism too small for the human eye to see unaided, especially a bacterium, virus, or fungus.

MOLECULE A particle formed when two or more atoms join together chemically.

MOTILE Able to move around.

MUCUS Thick, slimy fluid secreted by mucous membranes and glands for lubrication/protection.

MUTATION A spontaneous, permanent and hereditary change in the DNA sequence of a gene.

MUTUALISM A symbiotic relationship in which two organisms of different species live in a close association, each benefitting from the activity of the other.

NATURAL KILLER CELL A large white blood cell (or lymphocyte) that can destroy tumor cells and cells infected by viruses or bacteria.

NEUROTRANSMITTER A chemical messenger that transmits signals in the nervous system from one nerve cell to another, or to a muscle or gland cell.

NUCLEUS In eukaryotic cells a nucleus is typically a single, rounded, dense structure. It is bounded by a double membrane. The nucleus contains the cell's genetic material.

ORGANELLE A membrane-bound unit in the cytoplasm of a eukaryotic cell. Organelles perform specific functions essential to a cell's survival; examples are mitochondria or chloroplasts.

PARASITISM A symbiotic relationship in which an organism from one species (the parasite) lives in or on an organism from another (the host). The association benefits the parasite but is damaging to the host.

PATHOGEN A bacterium, virus or parasite that causes disease.

PENICILLIN An antibiotic originally obtained from certain blue molds but now usually produced synthetically.

PEPTIDE Between 2 and 50 amino acids linked in a chain. Peptides are smaller and less complex than proteins.

PERSISTER A bacterium able to survive a level of antibiotic that will kill almost all members of its species.

PH An indication of how acid or alkaline a solution is.

PLASMID A circular strand of DNA in the cytoplasm of bacteria. Plasmids can be acquired from viruses, other bacteria or the environment, and allow a bacterium to improve its performance.

POPULATION A group of bacteria of one species that interbreed and live in the same place at the same time.

PREBIOTIC A non-digestible food ingredient, usually plant fiber, that promotes the growth of beneficial gut microorganisms. Prebiotics act as fertilizers for the good bacteria that are already resident in the gut.

PROBIOTIC A supplement that introduces beneficial bacteria into the gut, often in the form of live bacteria in yogurt, other dairy products or pills.

PROKARYOTE A single-celled organism with no membrane-bound nucleus or other organelles: its genetic material (DNA) exists free in the cell. Bacteria and archaea are prokaryotes.

PROTEINS Basic structural components of all living organisms, consisting of long chains of amino acids (more than 50) folded into particular shapes. Proteins also function as hormones, enzymes and antibodies, all essential to the body's well-being.

PROTOZOA A single-celled eukaryotic organism. An example is the parasite that causes malaria.

RECEPTOR A molecule attached to a cell membrane. A receptor responds specifically to an interaction with a particular neurotransmitter, hormone or other biological molecule.

RESISTANCE FACTOR A genetic component of some bacteria that provides resistance to antibiotics. It can be transferred from one bacterium to another by conjugation.

RIBOSOME A complex structure in the cell cytoplasm that makes proteins.

SELF-PROTEIN A protein made by the body, to which the immune system should be tolerant. If the immune system malfunctions and recognizes the proteins as non-self, autoimmune diseases may occur.

SEPSIS A life-threatening condition that occurs when the body's immune system overreacts to an infection (anywhere in the body).

SEROTONIN A neurotransmitter involved in the transmission of nerve impulses. Often known as the "feel good" hormone, serotonin does play a key role in mood regulation and is also involved in the brain's perceptions of pain and the regulation of feelings of hunger and fullness in the gut.

SPECIES A group of closely related organisms very similar to each other; they are usually capable of interbreeding and producing fertile offspring. Applied to bacteria, "species" refers to a collection of strains with a common origin that are more similar to one another than to other strains.

STRAIN A genetic variant of a bacteria that is descended from a single bacterium. After mutating it is no longer a clone of the original bacterium, but is very closely related to the original species.

SUBCLINICAL INFECTION An infection that is nearly or completely lacking in signs or symptoms.

SYMBIOSIS A close, long-term association between organisms of different species. Forms of symbiosis include mutualism (benefit for both species), commensalism (benefit for one species, neutral for the other) and parasitism (benefit for one, damage to the other).

SYSTEMIC Affecting the whole body

T CELL A key lymphocyte (white blood cell) of the immune system. Helper T cells assist B cells to make specific antibodies against microbes. Cytotoxic T cells kill infected cells, while suppressor T cells keep immune responses under control.

VACCINE A vaccine is a killed or weakened form of an organism. When introduced to the body, it "trains" the immune system, stimulating the production of antibodies and cellular immunity without actually causing disease. The process of vaccination "trains" the immune system, preparing it for an encounter with a living form of that organism.

VIRUS A very small infectious agent that requires living cells in order to reproduce. Viruses reproduce inside the host's cell and damage it as they break out. They can infect animals, plants and also bacteria.

INDEX

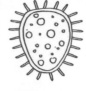

Page numbers in **bold**
indicate illustrations

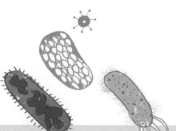

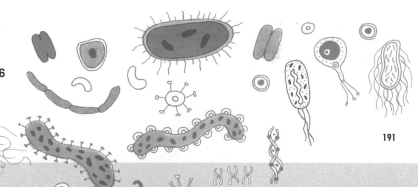

PICTURE CREDITS

Alamy Stock Photo BSIP SA 140r; Chronicle 47, 55; INTERFOTO 46; Edwin Remsberg 20; VintageMedStock 176b.
Getty Images BSIP/UIG 106b; Steve Gschmeissner/Science Photo Library 85, 140-141; Paul Hanny/Gamma-Rapho via Getty Images 180; Dr. Fred Hossler/Visuals Unlimited 122; National Institutes of Health/Science Photo Library 66; Alfred Pasieka/Science Photo Library 172b; Science Photo Library 172c. **iStock** duncan1890 43c, 44r; ibusca 44l; ivan-96 43l; Man_Half-tube 130; nicoolay 43r; photoka 137. **Science Photo Library** Dennis Kunkel Microscopy 77, 86t, 135; Dr. Kari Lounatmaa 59. **Shutterstock** Africa Studio 164; Sira Anamwong 156-157; AuntSpray 172t; Elena Baryshkina 119; Betacam-SP 70, 72b, 74t; Borisoff 158t; Rich Carey 158b; Cathal_Shtadler 168-169; cristovao 56; zu difeng 149; DiViArt 146; Ryazantsev Dmitriy 57tl; DoubleBubble 175r; Marco G Faria 145; Juan Gaertner 138-139; Oleg Golovnev 45r; ifong 136; Eric Isselee 140l; Iynea 42, 116; Rosa Jay 141r; johnjohnson 32-33; Jommar 41; Matej Kastelic 143b; Kateryna Kon 19, 25, 37 inset, 111, 125, 140-141, 143t; Komsan Loonprom 37; LightField Studios 76; Makc 68; MaraZe 61; marekuliasz 162; Morphart Creation 45l, 52, 73t, 78, 80, 87, 90-91, 93r, 100-101, 103, 174, 175l, 182-183; nobeastsofierce 13; Dmytro Novitskyi 114, 134; Oksana_Slepko 115; ostill 33; Pressmaster 57bl; rickyd 57tr; royaltystockphoto.com 8-9, 50; Aldo Santosa 179; David M. Schrader 154; Shai_Halud 24 inset; Sirirat 32; Slava_kovtun; Stocksnapper 156r, 183; Twin Design 45; Yuriy Vlasenko 23. **U.S. Centers for Disease Control and Prevention** 131; Janice Haney Carr 95; Medical Illustrator 75b, 86b; National Institute of Allergy and Infectious Diseases (NIAID); courtesy of Julie Marquardt 63. **Wellcome Collection** 93l, 106t, 128, 181; David Gregory & Debbie Marshall 105 S. Schuller 120.

FURTHER READING

Belkaid, Y. and Hand, T.W., 2014. "Role of the microbiota in immunity and inflammation." *Cell* 157(1): 121–41

Knight, R., "How our microbes make us who we are." *TED 2014*

Smith, P.A., 2015. "The tantalizing links between gut microbes and the brain." *Nature* 526: 312–314

Turnbaugh, P.J. et al., 2007. "The human microbiome project: exploring the microbial part of ourselves in a changing world." *Nature* 449 (7164): 804–10

Zhang, Y.-J. et al., 2015. "Impacts of gut bacteria on human health and diseases." *International Journal of Molecular Sciences* 16 (4): 7493–7519

Ames, Sebastian, *Bacteria: A Very Short Introduction*. Oxford University Press (2013)

Collen, Alanna, *10% Human: How Your Body's Microbes Hold the Key to Health and Happiness*. William Collins (2015)

Enders, Giulia, *Gut: The Inside Story of our Body's Most Under-Rated Organ*. Scribe (2014)

Madigan, Michael, et al., *Brock Biology of Microorganisms*. Pearson (2014)

Yong, Ed, *I Contain Multitudes: The Microbes Within Us and a Grander View of Life*. Bodley Head (2016)

For a full list of scientific papers, please see www.catherinewhitlock.co.uk and www.nicolatemple.com